DID I PACK MY STETHOSCOPE?

My Life As An In-Flight Nurse

Wendy Seddon

Copyright © 2021 Wendy Seddon

All rights reserved

Published in the United Kingdom

This book is dedicated to my parents, John and Clare. They taught me about courage and love and gave me a secure base from which to fly.

Per Ardua Ad Astra
(Through adversity to the stars)

CONTENTS

INTRODUCTION

Until I started working as an In-Flight Nurse I didn't have any idea what the role entailed. In fact, I'd never even heard of such a job. But what I did know was that the words 'In-Flight' and 'Nurse' used together gave me goose bumps. Could there possibly be a job where I could combine my nursing skills with my passion for flying and travel? Where I could do the things I loved and actually get paid for it? That's the dream for most people, and I was no different. If such a job existed then I wanted it.

Coming from an RAF family, a fascination for flying was within me from a very young age. My Dad's stories nurtured a passion that would last a lifetime and I hung on his every word, always wanting more. The desire to travel and to experience that sense of freedom and adventure just grew and grew like a pearl in an oyster growing from a grain of sand into something shiny and beautiful. I was inspired and motivated, and I wanted it more than anything.

But whilst growing up, I also developed a deep desire to care for people. Losing my sister, Andrea, when she was four, and watching my Mum look after her with such love and devotion, led to me pursuing a career in nursing. Doing a job that made a difference - easing suffering and helping people - became very important to me.

But there was also an element of survivor's guilt lurking within me. Why had Andrea died and I hadn't? It clouded my life growing up and I found myself constantly trying to make it up to my Mum; trying to fill the void that Andrea left. This, of course, was something I would never be able to do, but I didn't know that then, and it subsequently led to feelings of not being good enough. I yearned to make Mum happy and to make her proud of me. I hoped that becoming a nurse would do that.

Once qualified, I found myself in a profession that was both satisfying and rewarding. Working in a hospital proved interesting and challenging, and I quickly became skilled and experienced in Critical Care Nursing. But I knew this was just the start of my career; that I would not stay in one place for long; that there was more than just shift work and the daily commute.

But at this point I didn't know what that 'more' was. I had no idea that a role existed outside of the military where I could combine my two passions . . . until the day a two-line job advert in a magazine dangled the words 'In-Flight' and 'Nurse' in front of me. Eager to find out more, I rang the number immediately. The job involved flying abroad to bring people home who had been injured or taken ill whilst overseas. Sometimes it was with a doctor on the air ambulance but often it was travelling alone and bringing the patient back on scheduled commercial flights. It was my dream job. To my great surprise and delight, I beat 200 other applicants and the role was mine.

Friends expected me to spend my days jetting around the world, flirting with handsome pilots and dashing doctors, my nails painted and hair perfectly done. In short, the image was one of a glamorous, easy job. Or as one friend put it, "A glorified 'trolley-dolly'".

But, as is often the case, the reality proved to be somewhat different.

Most of the time it was a long way off being glamorous. And it most definitely wasn't easy. Exciting, thrilling, interesting it certainly was, but it could also be stressful, exhausting and sometimes downright harrowing. But it did send me on many incredible adventures, taking me to some stunning places and introducing a myriad of fascinating people along the way. From the outback in Australia to Kathmandu in Nepal; from seventeen-year-old rugby players to little old ladies with a passion for whisky; from whizzing through the jungle in a helicopter to making an emergency landing in the air ambulance at a French airbase. It was very different from what I expected it to be, but in a good way - even when my clothes were creased, I hadn't slept for 48 hours straight, and the last thing on my mind was whether my hair looked good.

Along the way there were times of brutal reality that challenged my confidence and taught me some hard lessons. But the job also showed me what true bravery looks like. From 28-year-old Ralph, fighting his way back from catastrophic brain damage, to Elsie, an old lady who quietly held her dead husband's hand after he passed away on a flight home from Africa.

Without a doubt, it was a thrilling and exciting period in my life.

Now, I'd like to share some of those adventures with you. Take you inside the world of an In-Flight Nurse, show you what goes on and what it's really like. Share the joys and the heartbreak, the thrills and the dangers.

Along the way I'd also like to give you an insight into my child-hood and the family that inspired me to make the choices I did. From my Dad who pushed his own dreams to one side to hold our family together after Andrea died, to my Mum who had the heart of a lion and taught me that love is the only thing that really matters. And also how I faced my own demons, eventually coming to terms with my past and moving forward to a positive and happy future.

I hope you enjoy the ride.

CHAPTER 1

Myrtle Beach

"One, two, three, four, five, breathe."

I don't know quite what I expected for my first trip as a fully qualified In-Flight Nurse, but it wasn't this. I was on my knees in the galley of a Heathrow-bound 737 doing cardiopulmonary resuscitation – CPR – on my patient who had been laughing and joking minutes before. His name was Frank, his heart had stopped, and he was in big trouble.

A doctor, responding to the call for medical assistance put out by the captain, had grabbed a face mask and was pushing air into Frank's lungs. I was doing chest compressions. Blankets, held up by two cabin crew, shielded us from the shocked eyes of the other passengers.

"One, two, three, four, five, breathe," I counted as I pumped on Frank's chest. He had been down three minutes. So far, no response to our efforts. Flat line. Every ticking second dragged us closer to losing him and hammered in my ears louder than the plane's engines. "One, two, three, four, five, breathe." My mind struggled to comprehend what had just happened. This couldn't be real. Had I missed something? Had the signs been there and I hadn't seen them? My shoulders began to ache as I continued on. "One, two, three, four, five, breathe." Still Frank's heart refused to do anything but flat line.

Just a short while ago things had been going so well.

Flying into Myrtle Beach, South Carolina, in the United States, it was my first job after getting my 'wings'. Excitement and trepidation swirled together in a heady cocktail of emotions with just a smidgen of fear floating near the top. In order to be as prepared as possible I had used the flight time to read the notes I had been given and go over in my mind what my plan was and what I would need to do. Travelling alone, I was acutely aware that the responsibility for the trip and my patient's wellbeing rested firmly on my shoulders. It was all down to me: every action, every decision, every problem would be mine. And I was an awfully long way from home which dialled up the intensity and made the cocktail fizz like a shaken up bottle of champagne. But I was trained and I knew what to do: this was my job now. It would be okay.

After 12 hours rest in a hotel, a taxi delivered me to the local medical centre to collect my patient, Frank. A gleaming, modern building greeted me, full of long corridors and big windows that bounced the morning light around like a series of mirrors. White uniformed nurses busied around and one very kindly directed me to Frank's room.

He had had an accident whilst on holiday with his wife and unfortunately had fallen very badly down a damaged drain cover. The momentum as he walked had propelled him forward onto his knees with his feet still trapped in the hole. Both his ankles had immediately snapped. Surgery had pinned the fractures back together and two plaster casts now protected his injuries, but he found himself unable to weight bear and needing a wheelchair to get about.

Fairly straightforward I was told; just do what's known as a 'handhold' and escort him home. Adjusting my rucksack on my shoulder, I took a deep breath and tapped on his door. Here we go, I thought, time to get the show on the road.

A tanned, well-built man with close-cropped grey hair, Frank gave me a huge smile as I walked in and introduced myself. It was obvious he was extremely pleased to see me as my arrival meant he was going home. An easy going manner and boyish laugh made me like him straight away although as we chatted I got the impression that the fall had shaken him up more than he was admitting to. His notes had told me he was a 52-year-old police sergeant which explained his bravado: he would be used to keeping his feelings under wraps and just getting on with things.

His wife, Ann, sat off to the side, framed by the blazing sun streaming through the big picture window. A petite lady dressed casually in jeans and a white blouse, she looked younger than Frank. A blonde bob framed gentle brown eyes and a shy smile touched her cheeks. She was also chatty and friendly but in a quieter more reserved way. However, she wasn't as good at maintaining the façade as Frank was: anxiety and tiredness etched her face with worry lines whilst dark circles smudged the skin beneath her eyes. Apart from her concern about Frank's injuries, she had also borne the stress of suddenly finding herself alone in such a vast country and having to handle all the formalities relating to Frank's care. However, relief brightened her face as she now realised she had someone to share the responsibility with. It felt good to know I was able to help them both and I breathed a sigh of relief that my first job would involve such nice people.

Of course, the cocktail of nerves was still sloshing around in my stomach. The skill was in putting forward a professional front that made it seem as if I had done this a hundred times before. I continued chatting away to put them both at ease and to keep me focused and busy. Many years spent working on NHS wards had taught me that this was a simple and effective tool that created a much calmer and relaxed environment for all concerned. It didn't matter the topic, just anything light hearted that built a connection and provided a distraction.

Ann packed the last of their possessions and I gathered Frank's case notes, x-rays and 'Fit-to-Fly' certificate. Everyone who had had surgery or been in hospital within the previous 14 days needed a form, signed by the treating doctor, to say they were fit to travel. Without it we would be denied boarding so it had been stressed to me the importance of checking this very carefully. Everything was in order.

Next job on my mental to-do list: check his observations. My shiny new blue stethoscope detected a slow, steady heart beat and a blood pressure that was within normal limits. His oxygen saturation levels were 100%. All good. A nurse named Becky came with pain killing medication for him and then we were ready.

A smooth ambulance ride got us to the airport in good time.

After our paperwork was cleared, we were joined by an airline customer care agent who pre-boarded us before the other passengers. The wheel chair we were using for Frank was too wide to fit onto the aircraft so he was transferred onto a smaller chair that was more like a sitting stretcher. This was much narrower and fitted easily through the door and down the aisle of the aircraft. Transferring Frank over to his seat was a little tricky, however, as Frank was six feet two and unable to bear any of his own weight on his injured ankles. It was lucky the repatriation company that I was working for had thoughtfully booked us assistance at the airport or I would have struggled on my own. The agent helped me to transfer Frank over and to get him settled. Bulk head seats at the front of the cabin gave us more leg room than standard seats but it still took a bit of effort manoeuvring him into position. Frank did his best to help us and we all sighed with relief when he was finally settled and comfortable.

The plaster casts on Frank's ankles had been bi-valved (cut down each side to make sure any swelling of his legs during the flight didn't cause them to become too tight and then restrict blood flow to his feet) and bandaged to hold them in place so I checked they were still in position and that the circulation to his toes was good. It was, so I moved on to checking his vital signs again: pulse, blood pressure and oxygen saturation levels. All remained good. The pain relief Frank had been given before leaving the hospital had kicked in so he was comfortable and in good spirits. The other passengers boarded, flight demos were done and we left on time. So far so good, I thought, settling back into my seat ready for the long flight.

Conversation flowed freely as we ate our meal. I learned they had two grown up sons, both at university, and that Frank was in fact a dog handler in the police. He became very animated as he told me all about his current dog, Hero, and what sorts of things they got up to when working a shift together. He described tracking car thieves and missing persons, doing raids on warehouses, and often ending up covered in mud when recovering stolen goods hidden in fields and bushes. It was obvious he loved animals and was in his dream job. Ann loved dogs too but admitted she felt a little jealous sometimes of the amount of time her husband spent with Hero. Although she then gave a little smile and went on to say she didn't really mind as she knew how happy it made him. I had to smile too when this big strapping policeman pulled a picture of his big tough police dog out of his wallet to show me; they were cuddling on an armchair like two big softies!

The in-flight movie came on - a romantic comedy that was easy watching and helped pass the time - and then the cabin lights dimmed and we settled back to rest for a while.

The cocktail of nerves in my stomach was beginning to lose a bit of its fizz. Although I was confident I could handle the job, I'd be lying if I said it wasn't a little bit scary. Many years in hospital critical care units had given me all the skills I needed to care for people but it was very different to be on my own with a patient so far from home and flying at 38000 feet without medical back up should it be needed. In a hospital you have a certain sense of security as you know you only have to pick up the phone and a doctor can be with you minutes later. But it was a 'handhold' job, so called because the patient wasn't ill as such, they just needed someone to metaphorically hold their hand and get them home. And it was all going nicely to plan.

Until suddenly it wasn't.

Frank started to get restless and to feel a 'little off'. He tried to play it down saying it was just 'indigestion' from eating his meal too quickly but I could see the colour draining rapidly from his face and a greyness washing over his skin. Sweat beaded on his forehead and when I held his wrist to check his pulse he was cold and clammy to the touch. Frank didn't want a lot of fuss but he let me do his blood pressure again and recheck his oxygen levels. Part of the kit that I carried with me was a small blood pressure machine, a stethoscope and a pulse oximeter which is a small, clip-like device that can be attached to a patient's finger to measure how well oxygenated they are. The readings of all his vital signs flashed dire numbers at me. Frank's pulse was fast, weak and thready, his blood pressure had dropped considerably and his oxygen levels were far too low.

By this time one of the cabin crew, a friendly red-headed young lady named Stacy, had noticed that something was wrong. She came over to see if she could help.

"Can you get us some oxygen?" I asked.

"No problem, I'll be right back."

True to her word she arrived back a minute later with a small bottle of oxygen with a face mask attached to it via a piece of clear tubing. Frank was struggling to breathe now so I quickly placed the mask over his face and turned the oxygen on full. For a couple of minutes it seemed to help and his breathing slowed a little. He was calmly taking deep breaths as I had asked him to, but his eyes, which were locked on me, were filmed over with fear.

And then he said, "I have pain across my chest."

My own heart metaphorically dropped. This was most certainly that last thing I wanted to hear when we were trapped in a metal tube flying over a vast ocean.

"What's it like?" I asked, gently reaching over and squeezing his hand.

"Like an elephant is sitting on me."

This was rapidly developing into a very serious issue. Thoughts of what to do next raced through my mind. Then suddenly, Frank started to make a loud snoring noise, his eyes glazed over and his head slumped forward onto his chest. I had heard that distinctive sound many times before and I knew immediately that when I checked his pulse there wouldn't be one.

He was in cardiac arrest.

Stacy, who had been standing to one side watching, rushed

off to get help. We had sat Frank in the aisle seat with me in the middle and Ann by the window so now I had to climb over Frank to get out. We needed to start resuscitation straight away. To do so we had to get Frank out of his seat and onto the floor. I struggled over into the aisle and started to pull Frank forward. Help came quickly in the form of two male cabin crew. They rapidly, and as gently as possible, got Frank onto the floor and pulled him into the galley area where we would have a little more room to work. As anyone who has ever flown on a commercial airliner will know, aircraft aisles are very narrow and difficult to move around in. There were also people sat immediately next to us, so all this was being played out in full view of the surrounding passengers. I glanced at Ann. Terror had frozen her in her seat, her eyes wide with the horror of what she was seeing. As I squeezed in beside Frank on the floor to begin CPR, I managed to make eye contact with Stacy; she nodded imperceptibly and I knew she had understood my silent request as she moved towards Ann.

Training and experience kicked in and I quickly cleared Frank's airway. One of the crew produced a red emergency bag and I heard the captain putting out a request for any doctors on board to make themselves known. Placing my hands one over the other, I locked my elbows and rapidly established a steady rhythm pushing down on Frank's chest; hard enough to be effective but not so hard as to break his ribs. On a fully grown man it takes a surprising amount of pressure to do chest compressions but I had done it many times before so knew how much force was needed. It is also crucial to do chest compressions fast enough as it has been proven that even when done perfectly, resuscitation only delivers a fraction of the normal amount of oxygen to a patient's brain. To give them even a small chance of recovery you have to be spot on; one of the reasons that CPR training in hospitals is so in-depth and involves a lot of practise.

One of the male cabin crew, who I later found out was called Mark, dropped to his knees at Frank's head and began using the Ambu bag – a face mask with inflatable bag attached – to start squeezing some oxygen into Frank's lungs. Protocols have changed now but then for every five chest compressions we would stop and give one breath. You don't do both at once as you would be working against each other and neither manoeuvre would be effective.

"One, two, three, four, five, breathe," I counted. "One, two, three, four, five, breathe."

I was vaguely aware of the cabin crew creating a screen around us with blankets and I was grateful for their thoughtfulness. Resuscitations can be very distressing to see as they can appear quite brutal, and I can only imagine how horrific it is to see someone you love having to go through one. I hoped Ann was still in her seat and therefore protected a little bit from the horror of what was happening to her husband.

As Mark and I continued working, a young man in jeans and t-shirt eased himself into the galley. He introduced himself quickly as Dan. Dan was a junior doctor who had responded to the call for assistance. He quickly knelt by Frank's head and took over with the Ambu bag.

We stopped briefly to check Frank for a pulse as I quickly filled him in on what had happened.

"No previous cardiac history?" he asked.

"No, a history of surgery three days ago to repair his fractured ankles but apparently fit and well otherwise."

"Any medication?"

"Just analgesia and antibiotics."

"Ok, let's get him connected to the defib."

The aircraft had a defibrillator on board which is a small machine that can be used to administer an electric shock to the patient if needed. It also had a screen on it that could be used as a cardiac monitor so that we could actually see what rhythm the heart was in. Two rhythms usually produce cardiac arrest: one is when the heart starts 'fibrillating' and the other is when it stops completely and you get the classic straight line. Fibrillation means the heart is firing lots of electrical signals which are chaotic in nature and don't produce a heartbeat – this is the kind of rhythm that responds to being given an electrical shock as it can reset the rhythm and start the heart beating properly again. It appears on the monitor as a jagged line. On the other hand, asystole or 'flat lining', doesn't respond to a shock and is the more serious of the two arrest situations. Unfortunately, on applying the sticky electrodes to Frank's chest and wiring him up to the defibrillator, this was the heart rhythm he was in. Giving him an electrical shock was pointless.

Dan grabbed a cannula from the emergency bag and managed to insert it into a vein in Frank's arm. He then rapidly injected a dose of adrenaline to try and stimulate the heart muscle. The monitor still flashed a flat line. We continued on with CPR.

"One, two, three, four, five, breathe."

I had been doing chest compressions for a while now and tiredness was beginning to creep up on me. Wedged in between Frank and the food trolleys, it was impossible to change position. Normally when resuscitating you would swap from one to the other so that the person doing compressions gets a break as it is such hard work.

Dan gave another shot of adrenaline and we stopped again to check for a heartbeat.

"Nothing," he said.

I caught his eye and the same thought passed between us. There was a very real danger that we were going to lose Frank.

"We need to give intra-cardiac adrenaline," I said.

Dan nodded.

Sensing that Dan was quite a junior doctor, I quietly asked, "Have you done it before?"

He shook his head.

Giving adrenaline directly into the heart muscle is a risky procedure especially if the person doing it is inexperienced, but at this moment in time we had run out of other options. The final thing in our arsenal, it was Frank's last chance.

Dan grabbed another syringe of adrenaline from the emergency bag and attached a long silver cardiac needle. I stopped chest compressions and sat back. Dan appeared calm and confident as he carefully felt between Frank's ribs. His hand trembling ever so slightly was the only outward sign that he was apprehensive. Finding the right spot, he slowly inserted the needle up to its hilt, drew back blood to make sure he was in the right place, and then steadily injected the 10mls of fluid. Straight into Frank's heart. Dan then pulled the needle out and sat back.

The watching cabin crew fell silent as we all stared at the tiny monitor sitting on the floor by Frank's head. Waiting.

I had a moment to register the enormity of what was happening. To think it was like something from a film. I couldn't believe I'd found myself in this position. That there was a very real chance that my laughing and cheerful patient could die on my very first job. What the heck had happened? Somewhere in the distance I heard sobbing and my heart ached for Ann having to see her husband like this. The plane's engines seemed to roar even louder in my ears and the smell of fish seeping out from the food trolleys made me nauseous. Death quietly edged her way out of the corner and stood breathing down my neck making my skin prickle and my breath catch in my throat.

One second, two seconds, three seconds, four seconds - please let this work - five seconds, six seconds . . .

And then there it was – a heartbeat! Then another and another. I slid my fingers to Frank's neck and checked for a pulse. There was an output. His heart was pumping again. Then he took a big gasping breath of air on his own.

Dan's face broke into a huge grin and I couldn't resist returning it with one of my own. We had had our own little miracle on a Heathrow bound jet at 38000 feet. Enormous relief washed over me as the cabin crew started clapping. Then all the passengers in economy joined in and started cheering. It really was just like a scene in a movie, except Frank wasn't an actor who would just get up when the director yelled 'Cut!' He was Ann's husband and he had children and a home and a job. And now, thankfully, he still had a life. I am not a religious person, but in that moment I silently thanked whoever had been watching over us.

A few minutes later the captain came to see us. We were thirty minutes away from landing at Heathrow. He had radioed ahead to arrange a team to meet us. In the meantime we agreed the best thing to do was leave Frank on the floor. It was far from certain that he wouldn't arrest again so we felt moving him into a seat was too risky. Dan graciously stayed with me to look after him. Pillows and blankets cocooned Frank to make him as comfortable and safe as possible and the cabin manager moved some of the other passengers so that Dan and I could have the two seats closest to the galley. The monitor continued to display a steady heart rhythm and Frank's respirations were slow and deep. His colour had improved but his skin was still waxy and pale and he had not yet regained consciousness. We stayed on our knees by his side until the very last minute then buckled up for landing.

I looked over at Dan.

"You did a great job there," I said. "Thank you so much for coming to help me."

He gave me a wry smile. "Truthfully, I was bricking it."

"How long have you been a doctor?"

"Two weeks."

"Ahh," I replied. "Well, I think you are going to be one damn fine clinician. You really kept your cool there."

"Thank you, I hope so. Childhood dream and all that."

"I was bricking it too," I admitted. "First trip as an In-Flight Nurse."

He glanced sideways at me. "What's one of those?"

I smiled. It was to be the first of many times over the coming years that I would get asked that question.

CHAPTER 2

Andrea 1968-1969

The day my sister Andrea died changed everything for my family. She was four and a half years old; I was six. Up until then my childhood had been safe and secure and happy.

Several years previously, my Dad, John, had joined the Royal Air Force Police. A posting to Laarbruch Airforce Base took us to Germany and home was a spacious house near the base with a wood at the bottom of the garden. An easy going manner combined with an ability to find the humour in just about any situation earned Dad lots of friends and our house often buzzed with the laughter and conversation of visitors. There was Corn-flake Bill, a young Australian with an obsession for that particular cereal; Klaus, who always arrived on his Heinkel scooter, blowing his horn and waving; and Carl, a big bear of a German man who Andrea and I adored as he always brought us sticky buns and marshmallows.

My Mum, Clare, was more quiet and reserved. Initially it was a real struggle for her to adapt to life in Germany. Making friends didn't come as easily as it did to Dad and loneliness snuck in and made her homesick. Sensing her sadness, two older German ladies who lived further up the street befriended her and kindly helped her to settle in. Firmly under their wing, they surrounded her in the maternal love she was missing, teaching her to bake bread and make delicious cakes. The aroma of her baking would fill the house making it feel warm and safe. Andrea and I spent many happy hours decorating her ginger biscuits with pink icing and smarties, and we loved sampling her sponge cakes just to make sure they had turned out ok.

Mum was in fact the complete opposite of Dad in just about every way. His outgoing, gregarious personality meant he got on with virtually everybody from cleaners to squadron leaders. Tall, with almost-black hair and blue eyes that crinkled with youthful mischief, he loved to be out and about and was always so full of energy that he ran everywhere. Mum, on the other hand, liked her own space and was happiest curled up with a book. They seemed to complement each other perfectly as Dad brought Mum out of her shell whilst she toned him down a bit. I guess there's some truth in the saying that opposites attract. Looking back at old photographs, they both seem impossibly glamorous with trendy clothes and sunglasses that were the height of sixties fashion. You tend to only see your parents as the older people in front of you when you are adult, but in truth, those old photographs are testament that Mum and Dad were far more glamorous in their hey-day than I have ever been or will ever be.

After settling into local life, there then came a Christmas that will forever be tucked away in my memories as a magical time that was so much better than any fairy tale I have ever read.

The German winter gifted us a wonderland of whiteness where fat snowflakes fell thick and fast as if our favourite marshmallows were falling from the sky. Wrapped up in our winter woollies, we pulled on our red wellington boots and crunched into the trees with Dad to build snowmen. Andrea and I were so small that sometimes we sank up to our waists in the soft snow, giggling and laughing as we tried to drag ourselves free. We never managed it. Dad to the rescue to haul us out and dust us down. Every now and then the cathedral of snow-laden branches above us would creak and groan and then dump great dollops of snow on our heads. It would stick to our eyebrows making us look like little old men whilst runny noses icicled our faces. The cold was biting and coloured our cheeks scarlet red, but it never bothered us as we were so busy building our creations: snowmen that were truly epic.

The best one we ever made we named Sammy. Round and solid, we piled up the snow as high as we could reach, our mittens never getting wet as the flakes were so dry and powdery and perfect. Dad lifted us up to finish off his head then we wound an old yellow scarf around his neck and pushed a carrot in for his nose. The finishing touch was big brown buttons for eyes that Dad produced with a wink and a flourish as if by magic from his coat pocket. Sammy was truly majestic as he held court over the creaking trees and whispering snow. On the way home we sang 'Frosty the Snowman' at the top of our voices, our words muffled by the white blanket that cloaked the trees and cocooned us from the rest of the world. Dad also had a cheeky packet of smarties in his magic pocket that he had slipped in when Mum wasn't looking. She would lecture him on the perils of giving us too much chocolate but he would just grin and make sure she didn't see him the next time he did it. It was a challenge to eat them with our mittens on but Dad would pop them into our mouths for us pretending they were tiny multi-coloured planes soaring back to base. Andrea got all the red ones as red was her favourite colour. The fact that her sweets matched her wellies delighted her.

Later that day, after it went dark, we headed into town to see the chapel and grottos sprinkled with hundreds of twinkling lights. Mum especially loved meandering slowly down the cobbled main street, taking in the smells of mulled wine and cinnamon buns that wafted from the shops. Everyone shouted to us and waved as we passed – some even thrusting sweets and biscuits into our hands. The evening came to a spectacular finale when we arrived at Santa's grotto to find it filled with a herd of live reindeer. Andrea and I gazed in wonderment as Santa presented each of us with a beautifully wrapped gift and then introduced us to two of his reindeer: Dasher and Dancer. Dasher licked Andrea on her ear and she squealed with delight, her blue eyes shining with happiness. She giggled with excitement all the way home as we walked hand-in-hand, clutching our presents and chattering away ten-to-the-dozen. It was ages before tiredness eventually caught up with us and Dad read us to sleep with a story of elves and their workshop buried deep in the snow at the North Pole.

The day after was Christmas Eve and it brought with it another whirl of excitement. Looking out of the window we felt as if we were in a snow globe as all the snow on the trees outside seemed to have been shaken up and was now falling again in great drifts and swirls. It mesmerized us, keeping us glued to the window for ages as we tried to count the flakes and watched Sammy, our snow man, disappearing under the swirling whiteness. Within an hour all that was left of him was the top of his head and the tip of his nose poking out like an orange full stop in the snow.

Darkness dropped early that day. We had a fabulous time sitting on the stairs together listening to Silent Night and Jingle Bells drifting up from the stereo. Having supposedly gone to bed in our new baby-pink nightdresses to await Father Christmas, we had crept down to spy on what was happening in the living room. Whispering and tittering quietly together we thought we were hidden from view but of course Mum and Dad could hear us. Dad made an extra special show of putting out carrots for Rudolph and a mince pie for Santa.

Christmas morning brought presents of all shapes and sizes wrapped in glittery paper and tied with red ribbon. Andrea's face broke into a huge grin when she opened one that contained an Andy Pandy glove puppet. With his smiling plastic face and blue and white striped cotton body, the puppet show on the television was her favourite thing to watch so she was thrilled even though she had bigger, more expensive presents.

In the corner, our Christmas tree towered over our pile of presents, its branches scraping the ceiling as if trying to burst through to the upstairs rooms. A golden angel glowed at the very top whilst baubles and fairy lights swathed it in twinkling reds and greens. Sweets dangled on golden threads, and paper chains that Andrea and I had carefully glued together ran colourfully through the green-ness.

Two days before, Cornflake Bill and Carl had appeared like yetis out of the swirling snow and taken Dad into the forest to get the tree. Tradition dictated that trees were freshly cut and carried back on the men's shoulders. Its glorious pine smell followed them into the house, bringing the forest to us and setting up a trigger that to this day whizzes me back to that moment. Mum laughing as they struggled to get it in the living room; Andrea and I giggling; the men trying not to swear as we kids were present. Dad insisted it had looked much smaller when it was in the forest but it was by far the biggest Christmas tree we ever had. Nature's glorious gift to us.

Cornflake Bill's family were all in Australia so he joined us for Christmas lunch. Dad cooked a feast of turkey and vegetables crowned with the best roast potatoes on the planet. Warm mulled wine flowed freely making the board games that followed great fun. There was chocolate log and mince pies, Quality Street chocolates and fruit cake, crisps and nuts. As Christmas Day trickled away into the night, Andrea and I fell asleep together in front of the fire with glowing cheeks and full bellies.

My memories of this time seem romanticised, like they have been lifted straight from the pages of a Hans Christian Anderson fairy tale. But that is how I remember it. Twinkly and shiny and perfect. I have no recollection of the icy pavements that threatened to throw you on your backside at every step, or the long nights cooped up in the house whilst Dad was on duty, or shivering away when the boiler broke and the pipes froze. To me it will always be a precious time frozen in a glittery, perfect snow globe. In essence, it's the only thing I have left of Andrea. For little did we know that it would be our last Christmas together. The following year we would be back in England and she would be dying.

Andrea had always been lauded as the quiet, well behaved one whilst I was the noisy and naughty tearaway. Then it became evident that she was quiet not just because she was well behaved but because she was ill. Cardiomyopathy was silently ravaging her body: a condition that causes the heart muscle to weaken and fail. Today it would have been picked up much sooner and she would have been listed for a heart transplant. Back then it went undetected until all her organs began to shut down one by one and she suddenly became very ill. By the time the doctors realised what was wrong, it was already too late.

The RAF showed great compassionate and understanding. When Dad's commanding officer found out that Andrea was so poorly he arranged for Dad to be posted back to the UK and we came home.

I remember clearly the evening that our GP, Dr Osman, came to my Nanna's house to see Andrea. An older Indian man with neatly-combed silver hair, he sat quietly listening to Mum tell him about how Andrea had been. A storm raged outside and as the November wind wailed down the chimney it brought with it a sense of fear and foreboding like something out of a Shakespearian tragedy. My young brain was too immature to understand the complexity of Andrea's symptoms but I knew that what was happening to her was very bad. With eighteen months difference in our ages, we weren't twins genetically, but in every other way we may as well have been. The same things made us laugh, we loved the same foods and games, and we did everything together. Now, her suffering became mine. I sat in the corner silently watching as Dr Osman gently carried out his examination. He took note of Andrea's swollen face and hands, her sallow skin, and the fact her breath was rattling in her chest like an old ladies. His sad eyes smiled gently at her as he stroked her hair and talked to her. Then he called an ambulance and arranged for her to be taken immediately to Bolton General Hospital.

Mum would not return home for the next 6 months. She stayed with Andrea in the hospital twenty-four-hours a day only going for a wash in the patient's toilets whenever Dad arrived to sit with Andrea. My Nanna looked after me. Sometimes Dad took me to visit Andrea – not often, though, as she was rarely well enough for me to go. In truth, I think it was more to protect me from seeing her in such a poorly condition. She was my soul mate, my best friend. I missed her with such ferocity I thought my heart would shrivel and die just like hers was doing.

Andrea's Andy Pandy puppet was her favourite possession and she kept it by her side the whole time she was in hospital. Until 3 days before she died.

Dad and I had gone to visit. We were met by a quiet and peaceful room with drawn curtains softening the morning sun into a haze of buttery light. Mum was in an armchair reading and Andrea was sleeping. We silently pulled up plastic chairs and sat down by her bed. Andrea's arm was resting on top of the covers and I was desperate to reach out and hold her hand but I didn't know if I should. I looked over at Dad and he seemed to sense what I was asking; he nodded gently. Reaching over, I carefully took Andrea's hand in mine; it was cool to the touch and swollen with fluid. After a few seconds I felt her squeeze my fingers and then her eyes fluttered open and she smiled at me. She pulled her other hand from beneath the blanket and in it was her Andy Pandy puppet. She held it out to me and said, "This is for you, Bendy." She could never pronounce the 'W' in my name so always called me 'Bendy'. It would be the last thing she ever said to me.

The day Andrea died is a day that lives permanently in a scar in my brain.

I heard it before I saw it: the latch on the back gate clicking open. I looked up to see Mum. In that instant I knew that Andrea had gone. Mum hadn't left her side for six months and would never have come home without her. It saddens me to remember Dad telling me later how they had come home on the bus from the hospital as they didn't have enough money for a taxi. To have to travel home on a packed bus when you have just lost your little girl – how desperately sad.

It was the 15th May 1969.

That day signalled the end of Dad's RAF career and changed the landscape of our lives in so many ways. But it was also the day that ignited a spark within me that would grow into a yearning to have a career caring for others as Mum had cared for

Andrea.

12 years later I started my nurse training and then got a job on the children's ward in Bolton where Andrea died. The senior sister on the ward, Sister Hartley, called me into her office on my first day and asked me if I was Andrea's sister.

"Yes," I said. "How did you know?"

"I never forget any of my children," she replied with a sad smile.

But as my career was forming, Dad's was ending and so too were his dreams of working with planes and travelling the world. Mum plunged into a deep, grief-induced depression and Dad knew it was time to be at home with his family. After being stationed in Germany, Dad had hoped to be posted further afield and to be around planes for the rest of this working life. Air Force life had immediately grabbed him, playing to his strengths and giving him a passion that filled him with enthusiasm. But he realised it wasn't the type of life that was suited to a newly bereaved family so he came out on compassionate grounds and went to work on 'civvy street'.

As we had lived in married quarters provided by the Air Force, coming out meant we had nowhere to live. My Nanna, Mum's mother, had graciously allowed us to live with her in her two-up-two-down terraced house when we returned to the UK from Germany. But it was tiny and cramped; there was no bathroom, only an outside toilet. It was a difficult and sad time for my parents.

Dad got a job in a wiring factory and worked long hours to provide for us. But in the evenings he would sit with me at the kitchen table and tell stories. Lots and lots of stories. They would always involve planes and flying and adventures. His words carried me to China and Africa and The Amazon. There were Vulcan bombers and daring rescues, dashing pilots and deadly missions into the jungles of Borneo. A gifted artist, Dad would draw pictures to illustrate the tales he told. I relished every word and became captivated by the idea of flying, exploring and seeking out new adventures.

Looking back I realise what a wonderful gift he gave me by

doing this. His stories protected me to a certain extent from the grief that suffocated our house whilst at the same time giving me a real sense of adventure. I was inspired to dream big, to be brave and to go after what I wanted.

CHAPTER 3

Kathmandu

My second trip abroad came at just the right moment. The phone rang at 10 am on a rainy Tuesday morning five days after I got back from South Carolina. Frank had been on my mind all week and I needed to both find out how he was and to have another job to distract me from going over every single detail of what had happened with him. I knew I had cared for him to the very best of my ability but I still couldn't shake the niggle of wondering if I'd missed something. And I suppose it was a bit like the old saying about riding a bike and the need to get straight back on if you fall off. My first job had gone horribly wrong so I needed to get straight back up and go again to prove to myself that I could actually do the job and do it well. I picked up on the third ring.

Before Julie from the office could say anything other than 'Hello', I cut her off.

"How's Frank?"

There was a pause of maybe two seconds but it was long enough for dread to grab my stomach and throw it down to my feet as I braced myself for bad news. But then, to my enormous relief, she replied, "He's doing well and is almost ready to go home."

After being admitted to hospital in London, it was found that a massive blood clot had blocked his main coronary artery causing a Myocardial Infarction or 'heart attack'. This had resulted in a large part of his heart muscle being deprived of oxygenated blood which had in turn then caused his heart to stop. Surgeons had managed to bypass the blockage and restore blood flow to the muscle but the damage had been considerable and by all accounts he was exceedingly lucky to have survived.

Whenever you resuscitate someone who has gone into cardiac arrest you automatically switch into professional mode, pushing your feelings to one side and concentrating on a strict protocol of actions to try and bring them round. Afterward though, it can hit you hard. When the event is finished, if it has a good outcome, it is enormously satisfying and uplifting. You know you have helped to save a life, you have made a very real difference, and a family has their father, husband, grandmother or sister back again. The opposite outcome can be very traumatic. Although you do get used to coping when a patient dies of a cardiac arrest, each loss takes a little piece of you with it. And sometimes you can't help but feel that you failed the patient. Could you have done more? Could you have done anything differently? And you can empathise with their family's pain and imagine what it would be like if it was your loved one. Cardiac arrests are so sudden, so abrupt, and having someone thumping up and down on your chest is an awful way to spend your last few minutes. As a nurse, you know people are relying on you and need you. You act as you are trained to but afterwards you can be left drained and emotionally rung out. And this particular situation had been ramped up significantly for me with it being my first repatriation and my first experience of resuscitating someone outside of a hospital environment. It was fair to say that I had been left drained and emotionally rung out.

But Frank had made it. It was a great outcome for us all and I was relieved and happy. And ready for my next job.

"Can you get to the airport by 4pm?" asked Julie.

She was the office manager at the repatriation company I worked for and the one responsible for booking flights, accommodation, stretchers, ambulances – basically anything that would be needed to get a patient safely back to the UK. A Welsh lady in her forties, she had a calm, organised manner about her with a soft and soothing voice that would have made her an excellent nurse if she had chosen that route. At this stage I didn't know her very well but I was already getting a sense that she was someone who could be trusted to look after as much as she could to facilitate a smooth repatriation and to do her best to help you if you encountered problems.

I looked at my watch: it was 10am. Plenty of time I thought.

"Yes, of course," I replied, eager to find out where I would be heading to.

And then she said, "Heathrow."

As I live just outside Manchester, which is a good 4-5 hour drive from Heathrow with traffic, it would be tight. I literally would have to grab my bag and leave immediately to make the flight. I learned very quickly to always have my rucksack packed and ready to go as it transpired that many of the jobs were 'Drop and Go' where I had to literally drop everything and go to the airport. It was most definitely not a job for people who liked everything organised and planned in advance, and would be very difficult for people with families or commitments. I was lucky as I had no responsibilities at that point and could just drop and go. I did however end up with no social life. Plans were made to see friends only to be cancelled at the last minute when a job came through. Luckily, my friends were understanding and didn't let it faze them, but I did give away quite a few theatre and concert tickets!

Travelling light was also something I learned to do right at the beginning of my In-Flight career. A small purple rucksack carried just one change of clothes and enough toiletries for a couple of days. Most of the jobs were a quick turnaround so that was enough. Having few personal items was essential as I often had medical equipment to carry or a patient in a wheelchair who also had bags to see to. If encumbered with a large bag of my own it would be very hard work. The problem came if I got stuck anywhere, which happened a few times, as I had little with me. Luckily my company was very good and just told me to buy whatever I needed and they then reimbursed me.

So, on a cold and grey winter's morning, I grabbed my bag,

said a hasty goodbye to my Mum and Dad, and headed off down the M6. My destination this trip was Kathmandu in Nepal. The fact that when the phone rang I never knew where in the world I would be headed was one of my favourite aspects of the job. It could be Ireland or France, or it could be Cape Town or Sydney. But today it was Kathmandu and a cloud of anticipation raced down the motorway with me.

Kathmandu was a bit of an unknown to me at the time. I knew it was the capital of Nepal, was the starting point for many Everest expeditions and that it was near India. But that was it really. I resolved to read up as much as I could whilst travelling in order to make the most of the trip.

Obviously, my focus on these jobs was always my patient, but often I would have a little free time before collecting them from the hospital. I would always make the most of this and try and see as much as I could of my destination. Luck was on my side too, as the repatriation company was a good one and they always booked me a nice hotel to stay in – nothing fancy but always pleasant and in a nice part of town. They also paid for meals. This meant I could explore areas and try different places to eat, confident in the knowledge I had a safe, secure base.

Most of the time the jobs were solo trips where I travelled out on my own using commercial flights. Only occasionally was a patient so ill that a doctor accompanied me and/or we would use the air ambulance. Travelling to such far-flung places alone did demand a certain amount of courage and confidence, and it wouldn't be for everyone, but I was quite happy. Whether this was just the naivety of youth I don't know but I rarely found myself dwelling on what could go wrong from a travel perspective. I had often travelled for pleasure on my own and was used to it. The sense of adventure and freedom was thrilling.

Many times over my career I visited the countries Dad had told me stories about and it was exciting to actually see the places for myself. Conjured up pictures of what they would be like often didn't match the reality: sometimes they were way better and sometimes a bit of a disappointment like the time I went to the pyramids in Egypt and there were fast food outlets near the Sphinx. And, of course, it was exciting to be able to turn the tables and tell Dad stories about the things I had seen and done; to bring all these exotic places to life for him as he had done for me all those years ago at our kitchen table. Our bond grew deeper because of it; a real shared joy. And, of course, there was always lots of discussion about which types of plane I had flown on.

The patient I was collecting this time was a female climber named Alice. Part way up Everest she had slipped and fallen about fifteen metres after some of her equipment failed. A ridge of rock had luckily broken her descent and stopped her falling much further. But she was injured. The jagged edges of the rocks had broken three of her ribs which had then punctured her lung on the left side. Air lifted off the mountain, she had spent several days in hospital where she had needed a chest drain inserted to drain the air from her pleural cavity and re-inflate her collapsed lung.

Approaching our destination the atmosphere in the cabin suddenly began to crackle with anticipation, almost as if someone had plugged the plane into a mains socket and the electricity was jumping from one person to the next. We were still flying above the clouds when to the left of the aircraft a snow-covered pinnacle of rock came into view, roaring up and into the blueness. Puzzled by the excitement of my fellow passengers, I didn't immediately click what it was until I heard someone whisper: Everest. Despite never having been interested in climbing, the sight captivated me. The sense of awe that she inspired had an almost magical element to it and everyone on board fell silent, transfixed by the view through the window. It was easy to understand the thrill of the people who were going to climb her. What a feeling it must be to actually stand on the top of that beauty knowing that you were at the very top of the world. I wouldn't ever do that but I felt extremely privileged to have seen her.

Arrangements had been made for Alice and me to fly out together the following day but I decided to go to the hospital to meet her and fill her in on the plans that had been made before I checked into my hotel. I was hoping for a smooth trip home this time with none of the drama of my first trip.

Expecting her to still be quite poorly, I was pleasantly surprised as I walked into her room. Sitting up in a chair, Alice chatted away with no breathing problems, a healthy glow to her skin and stable vital signs. A tough, adventurous lady – to be expected, I suppose, as she had been climbing the world's tallest mountain – she seemed fitter than me. We hit it off immediately. She told me she was a twenty-four-year-old veterinary student from Newcastle with a passion for outdoor sports – climbing in particular. Attempting Everest had been part of a charity challenge to raise money for a local dog rescue centre – a place that meant a lot to Alice as she had volunteered there since being a teenager. Disappointment that she hadn't completed the climb dripped from her words but she vowed to return and try again.

Despite Alice appearing so well she had still suffered a pneumothorax so we would need to be mindful of her breathing and oxygen levels on the flight. Extra oxygen had been booked in case she needed it and I had my pulse oximeter with me to keep an eye on her saturation levels as we travelled. Alice only had a few things with her but we packed them up ready then arranged I would come back for her the next day at 11am.

After a quick phone call to the airline desk to confirm our tickets and flight times, the rest of the day was then free for me to do so some exploring. I headed out of the hospital with a spring in my step despite the long flight I'd just done.

Kathmandu was unlike anything I had ever experienced before never having travelled in that part of the world. The cacophony of noise was the first thing that hit me closely followed by the vibrant, clashing colours and the obvious desperate poverty. Children were using the side of the road as a toilet and several were having a wash – naked - under a hose pipe. 'Shops' lined the road but I use the term loosely – they were in fact little more than crumbling piles of rubble with a few food items stacked on plastic tables in front of them. It was very much like I imagined India would be: traffic, bikes and people all competing for space in the crowded, dusty streets. A real eye-opener of a place that rammed itself down your throat right from the minute you arrived. I found it a little un-nerving at first but I quickly jumped into the thick of it and set off on foot to find my hotel and drop my bag off before doing a little sightseeing.

Great big orange trucks thundered past me blasting their horns and creating great clouds of dust that billowed behind them like dirty parachutes. Motor bikes that looked about two hundred years old weaved in and out around the children and I expected any minute to hear screams as one of them ran over a child. Amazingly, they all seemed to dodge around one another with seemingly few serious mishaps. Several pushbikes nearly careered into me before my hotel thankfully appeared across the road. But crossing over that road was another matter entirely. I waited patiently for a safe gap in the traffic but one never materialised. Eventually, I had to take a deep breath and run for it. It was lucky I had found the hotel at all as there were few road signs or name plates anywhere, but it was an absolute miracle I made it there alive across that road. What a dance with danger - it made crossing our city streets seem positively sedate in comparison.

Walking into the cool, air-conditioned lobby with gleaming marble floors and huge ornate vases full of pink orchids, the grandness contrasted sharply with the heat and dirt of the outside. Once the doors swished shut behind me, the noise of the street vanished and it was as if I'd entered a painting where everything was bright and polished and perfect with every detail carefully thought of and added in with exquisite skill. Such rich sumptuousness was hard to comprehend when only a few yards away in the street the children had no shoes and no toilets.

"Hello," said the smiling Nepalese lady behind the desk. "Are you Wendy?"

"Yes," I replied, somewhat confused. How on earth did she know who I was?

"We've been expecting you. Please, I would like to introduce you to Mendip."

"Ok," I said warily, "But who is Mendip?"

"Your guide."

Now I was extremely puzzled. My guide? The office seemed to take good care of us when we were travelling on a job but I didn't think that would extend to booking me a tour guide. It turned out that it was Alice who had very kindly arranged it for me. She had taken a tour with Mendip herself on first arriving in Nepal so after I left the hospital she had called him to see if he was free to take me out for the rest of the day. I had told her the name of my hotel so he had agreed to meet me there. This was not only extremely thoughtful of Alice but also quite amazing that he was there waiting for me – it was barely half an hour since I had left the hospital.

Mendip's grin was quick and genuine; his manner quiet and polite. He appeared young; maybe eighteen or nineteen, with short jet-black hair, and blue trousers that were just that little bit too short for his slim, six-foot frame. He bowed and then presented me with a cream silk prayer scarf. "For you," he said, placing it gently around my neck. His kindness was touching and I quickly warmed to his youthful charm.

"I will show you my city if you like," he said shyly after shaking my hand.

"I would like that very much," I replied. What a wonderful stroke of luck. I would see so much more with a guide than I could ever hope to see on my own with such limited time available. I was also quite relieved that I would have someone with me as the frenetic energy and chaos of the streets was a little bit overwhelming.

After a quick freshen up in my room, I found him patiently waiting for me in reception.

First stop was Swayambhunath, the Buddhist Stupa, festooned with multi-coloured flapping prayer flags. A stunning domed white building gilded with gold, it stood glittering in the sun at the top of a hill overlooking the Kathmandu valley. The gigantic painted eyes of the Buddha watched me as I gasped my way up the steps to the top. Kathmandu stands at 1400 metres above sea level so the air is a bit 'thin' and without time to acclimatise it was hard work. But goodness, it was worth it. The whole of the city stretched out before me and I truly felt on top of the world. Close up, the magnificence of the temple was even more striking. Built over two thousand years ago, both Hindus and Buddhists worship there. Prayer wheels were set into the ancient stone walls at regular intervals and I marvelled at their intricate designs as my fingers gently spun them around. It was awe inspiring to think of the many ancient hands that had touched them before me. Tucked away in a corner sat a tiny shop with a monk in burgundy robes sitting cross legged in front of a table loaded with beautiful, handmade wooden carvings. He patiently waited as my gaze travelled slowly over his wares, finally settling on a small elephant to take home for Mum.

And there were monkeys - lots of monkeys: big ones and little ones, adults and babies, some grooming each other, others racing across the walls and paths in a manic game of chase. Mendip found it hilarious when I sat down on a wall to have a breather and one of the little rascals stole my bottle of water!

Colourful markets came next, their stalls showing off all manner of trinkets and clothes. It was great fun to mingle with the crowds of locals fishing about in piles of goodies for more treats to take home. They had to be small, of course, as I couldn't carry much in my rucksack but that seemed to add to the pleasure of choosing. A blue cashmere scarf with the softest, most luxurious feel to it cost me the equivalent of three pounds. Wondering deeper into the market, spices and incense created a fragrant cloud that was heady and beguiling. I breathed it all in trying to fix the moment into my memory.

Then we were on the move again, heading to the Baghmati River and another temple, this time one revered by Hindus. The Pashupatinath temple stands right by the river and is completely different to Swayambhunath. Created in the style of a pagoda, its silver walls and gold roof reflected the sun in a dazzling display of brilliance. Considered a holy place by Hindus, cremations often take place on the banks of the river just down from the temple itself. Amazingly, one was just starting as we arrived. A little morbid you might think, and at first I was very unsure about watching as it felt intrusive, but the ritual, the funeral pyre, the incense were mesmerizing and it was humbling to join the crowds paying their respects to the deceased. I found myself holding my breath in reverence. It was deeply moving and felt like a true celebration of a life well lived. Mendip told me it was a lady who had been a wife, mother, grandmother and sister. We watched as white flowers floated on the water whilst candles, burning all along the river bank, gave off a flickering glow through the hazy smoke of the burning pyre. There was no mistaking how loved she had been. It struck me that to be loved in such a way is the true meaning of success in life.

Eventually we had to pull ourselves away as the sun melted into the water and darkness crept in along the river. The day was almost over and it was time to eat. And although I didn't think it possible, that was when my day became even more surreal. And surprisingly scary.

Thudding in my ears, my heart was beating so fast I feared it would explode out of my chest and land on the floor at my feet. Mendip was leading me down yet another pitch-black back alley. I was seriously wondering if at any moment I was going to be kidnapped or maybe even murdered. He was striding out in front of me, taking one turn and then another, holding a red plastic cigarette lighter out in front of him. Its tiny beam provided the only flicker of light in the otherwise solid wall of blackness in front of us.

I was cursing myself for having made such a serious mistake. It's only my second trip and I've done something incredibly stupid, I thought. I'm down a deserted alleyway in Kathmandu, at night, with a man I only met a few hours ago – how stupid could you be? The calm peacefulness that had settled over me after being at the river had fled. Now, my nerves were screaming at me to turn and run. To get away from this place as quick as I could. But I knew I couldn't. I had no idea where we were or how to get back to the safety of the main street. I didn't really have much option other than to keep following Mendip. To hope that he was as genuine as he had seemed; that he wasn't leading me into a horror story.

"Not much further now," he said, turning and flashing me a smile that appeared ghoulish in the beam of the flickering lighter. Oh gosh, please let this be ok.

I forced myself to take a deep breath and try to relax. He was supposedly taking me to a 'small, family-run restaurant' for our evening meal. I hoped and prayed that this would indeed be the case, but how on earth could these back alleys in the middle of nowhere be the home of a restaurant.

Another couple of anxious minutes thudded by. Uneven ground littered with stones and rubble tried to trip me up so I had to concentrate on not falling flat on my face in the blackness. It felt like if I went down that would be it. I would be engulfed and gone. Swallowed by the blackness of a Kathmandu night. My heart thundered on and my mouth was as dry as I could remember it ever having been.

And then a pool of light appeared ahead of us like the northstar guiding us in. Mendip homed in on it and I stumbled after him through a small rickety gate and into the 'restaurant'. What it was in fact was someone's back garden. By the side of the small wooden fence stood a white plastic garden table with four plastic chairs arranged around it. The light was a tiny, battery-powered lamp that stood by the table casting very welcome buttery yellow light across four basic place settings: a tiny folded piece of white cotton, a fork and a plastic tumbler at each.

The wooden gate creaked shut behind us triggering the appearance of two elderly people – a man and a woman. Both tiny and stooped, both obviously very old, but both wearing beautiful beaming smiles. The old lady shuffled slowly out of the darkness and over to me. Her hand reached out and took hold of mine, squeezing it gently and pulling me towards the table. The man had a jug of something in his hand and he started filling the tumblers.

Mendip was grinning as he clicked the lighter flame off and sat down at the table.

"Come, come," he said, "sit down and we will eat."

I was so relieved to be actually sitting down to a meal, even if it was at a plastic garden table, that it took me a minute to control my nervous laugh and think of something coherent to say. Fear had frozen my brain and my dry mouth had seized up my tongue. The best I could come up with was a lame "Sounds good."

It turned out that the tour company that Mendip worked for regularly used this little stop off as an authentic place for their guests to eat. Well, it certainly was authentic, even if getting to it was somewhat surreal and scary. But the food was good – a spicy lentil dahl with naan bread for dipping served on white paper plates. The old lady was attentive and kind and kept patting my hand as I ate whilst the old gentleman kept filling my tumbler with a sweet-tasting, syrupy juice that reminded me a little bit of mango but I wasn't sure if that was what it actually was. Neither of them spoke English so conversation was stilted as Mendip translated backwards and forwards.

After finishing my meal, I asked to use the toilet. Mendip gave me his lighter and pointed me out into the darkness. I edged out of the gate and found the 'toilet' was a hole in the ground hidden behind a three-foot wall. With no idea what was lurking in the undergrowth I decided to wait until I got back to the hotel. It's surprising how the threat of creepy crawlies and slithery things can dry up your bladder. The meal ended with a cup of weak tea without milk poured into our tumblers. Then, after hugging us both, the old couple waved us off into the darkness and once more I was trailing behind Mendip and his flickering lighter flame. I have to say that although they seemed genuinely lovely people and the food delicious, it is not an experience I want to ever repeat.

Once safely back at my hotel, Mendip dropped a bombshell. He said that the guides always took guests to the old couple because they were his grandparents and they had no other income or way to support themselves. He then added that they would not have eaten themselves the day before in order to save the food for guests. They had charged me the equivalent of £2 for my meal. I was so upset. I tried to give him more money for them but he wouldn't accept it. Bowing again, he shook my hand and then vanished out into the night.

Such a range of emotions assailed me it was hard to make sense of them: guilt for having eaten their food; shame for having been scared; sadness for the position they found themselves in. I felt lucky to be so privileged in life, to have never known anything but a full belly and a safe home. And I felt immensely grateful to have met Mendip and his beautiful grandparents. They had been so welcoming, so gracious and, amazingly, so happy. I will never forget the old lady's smile and her warm hands guiding me to her table. It was my first real introduction to the abstract poverty that exists in some countries around the world, and one that affected me profoundly.

My sightseeing day was over and I was exhausted but sleep eluded me that night. Images of funeral pyres and dark alleyways crowded my mind and by the time morning came I felt wiped out. But I had a job to do so had to get moving. A cold shower and two cups of coffee revived me and I headed out bright and early to collect Alice.

The day was blisteringly hot, the kind that makes you tired before you've done anything, and it was only 8am so likely to get much hotter. Dust and heat hazed the streets as I set off into the mayhem, narrowly missing a bright blue motorbike that screeched past me as I stepped out of the hotel.

Alice was dressed and ready and we set off for the airport with plenty time to spare before our flight. We were heading to Alice's home in Newcastle via Amsterdam and Dublin so a long day of travelling lay ahead of us. The crowds I'd come to expect greeted us at the airport like a rugby scrum. We had to elbow our way through to the airline desk to collect our tickets, taking care not to get separated in the crush. It seemed half of Kathmandu was flying out of this small airport all at the same time.

"There are no tickets here under that name," the agent said, clicking away on his computer without looking at us. He was tall with the same black hair as Mendip, but none of his charm.

"What?" I replied in puzzlement. "I rang yesterday and confirmed they were waiting for us."

He rapidly clicked more keys on his computer. "I'm sorry, there are no tickets here under that name."

I gave him Alice's name just in case the names had got mixed up and they'd been booked under her name instead of mine.

An impatient shake of the head. "Sorry, nothing."

Our tickets had been confirmed as waiting for us. What was going on? (This was before the days of e-tickets and emails to just print out.) The queue of people behind us was growing longer by the minute. The next in line, a man in a crumpled grey suit, pushed forward and jostled us away from the desk. Ok, I needed to ring the number I had rung the day before to find out what had happened to our tickets.

Hunting for a phone was a challenge but eventually Alice spotted one hidden in a far corner by a newspaper stand. A well-spoken lady picked up after one ring and assured me our tickets were there. Then the penny dropped. She had answered the phone with the name of a travel agency. Our tickets were ready and waiting for us, just not at the airport.

"Where are you based?" I asked.

She gave me the address then went on to say it was a twenty minute car ride from the airport – right across the other side of the city. We were going to be very pushed for time to get across town and back again in time for our flight but we had no option – without our tickets we couldn't fly.

Stifling heat slapped us in the face as we rushed outside as if trying to make things even more difficult for us. I scanned for a taxi.

"There, on the left," I shouted to Alice above the roaring of a departing plane.

Jumping in the back of a dirty green sedan I hurriedly gave the address to the driver and we hared off in search of our tickets. I glanced sideways at Alice. She had only just been discharged from hospital and the heat and dust were ferocious – not good for someone who had had a punctured lung only a few days ago - but she just smiled at me and said it was all part of the adventure. I was grateful that she was coping alright physically and really appreciated her positive attitude. It rubbed off on me and we were soon laughing like teenagers at the absurdity of it all.

Tickets in hand the taxi did an abrupt about turn and raced us back to the airport. It was supposed to be an easy going morning with no rush and plenty of time to make our flight. Instead it was like the wacky races as we careered around bikes and pedestrians, bumped over huge pot holes in the road and narrowly avoided a head on collision with a bright blue bus covered in prayer flags. I soon realised the best plan was to not watch the road – it was far too hair-raising! Our driver seemed to relish the challenge and we screeched to a halt back at the airport with thirty minutes to go before boarding for our flight closed. It would be a close call but we would make it.

By the time we sank into our seats on the aircraft we were sweaty, grimy and exhausted. Bottles of water that we had grabbed on the way through tasted like nectar even if they were rather tepid!

After a few minutes I managed to gather my thoughts and set about checking Alice's oxygen level with my oximeter. I was relieved to see it was fine at 98%. Her pulse and blood pressure were also good and most importantly, she was still in good spirits and chatting away. Travelling in Asia for a while had obviously seasoned her and she knew this kind of thing was par for the course and to be expected. She just rolled with the punches. It was another valuable lesson for me: on future trips I always made sure I had my tickets in hand or knew exactly where they were before collecting my patient.

The early days were a steep learning curve and it soon became apparent that many of the problems I would encounter would be logistical not medical. Airlines and airports are understandable very strict with the rules and they had to be followed precisely. Paperwork had to be spot on with all the required boxes ticked or they wouldn't let you fly. This could be checked carefully and planned for but of course other things happened unexpectedly. Ambulances/cars broke down, flights were cancelled, oxygen bookings had not been put through. You had to become very adept at thinking on your feet and finding creative solutions to problems, always putting the patient's welfare at the heart of everything. I also soon realised that it was essential to always have two credit cards on me with big credit limits. When on a job, I usually had to pay for things that were needed and then claim the money back when I got home. And sometimes the things needed were very expensive. I once had to upgrade myself and my patient to Business Class because she needed to have a reclining seat to elevate her swollen leg. Economy seats had been booked for us but weren't suitable. As we were in Barbados, it cost £2500 each – a total of £5000. Luckily I just had enough available on my card but from then on I always took two cards with at least £10000 just in case. There was never any problem claiming it back, and I was usually reimbursed within a few days, but I did have to lay it out in the first place.

Our flight continued on to Amsterdam without incident and we changed planes at Schiphol onto our flight to Dublin. And this was where we got a lovely little surprise treat. Alice's friend, as it turned out, was a pilot based in Dublin. He had found out which flight we were on and arranged for us to be upgraded. We both thoroughly enjoyed being spoiled and fussed over although sadly I couldn't partake of the free champagne as I was on duty.

As we journeyed, the conversation flowed on. Alice was warm and friendly and outwardly calm and relaxed, but the more she talked the more it became obvious that she was hiding her true feelings. Inside she was struggling. She told me how she had genuinely thought she was going to die on Everest when she fell. Coldness had invaded her body quickly and it had taken a long time for the rescuers to get to her due to where she was lying. Unable to move, starved of oxygen and in terrible pain, she had started to hallucinate. Vivid flashes of continuing to fall and then being entombed in the snow had overtaken her. She saw herself trapped in a white coffin, suffocating and dying. She described screaming and screaming to make them understand she wasn't dead and then fighting the rescue team with all her might as she thought they were then trying to bury her alive.

Once off the mountain and receiving treatment in hospital, the hallucinations had gone but she was plagued with flashbacks that set her heart pounding and drenched her in cold sweat. Several times a night she woke up in abstract terror, reliving the feeling of being buried alive as if it had really happened.

It was obvious she was suffering from Post-Traumatic Stress Disorder and was going to need expert help to get it under control. Over an hour passed as she talked about it. I sat and listened quietly, hoping it helped her to tell someone how she was feeling. She was trying so hard to keep it all together and put a brave face on.

It really brought it home to me that day that you do not know what suffering people might be keeping hidden behind a smile and a cheerful laugh. A brave front can hide so much. During nurse training we were always taught to see the patient as a whole and not just think of what condition they were being treated for but listening to Alice made it much more immediate and personal. Her story turned up the dial and made me much more aware of treating the whole person rather than just their illness or injury. Alice's medical problem was her lung/rib injury but her psychological trauma was causing her far more problems and needed just as much care and attention in order to help her get well again.

Making an effort to get to know my patients was always important to me but from that day on I made sure to always provide an opportunity for people to talk if they wanted to, realising more than ever the value of a listening ear if it was needed. This was much easier to do when working with patients on a one-to-one basis than it was in a hospital setting when you had lots of patients to think about. Sometimes people just needed to be heard, to feel that someone cared enough to listen. From my point of view it was tremendously satisfying to feel I was helping people get through what was obviously a very stressful event in their lives, compounded by the fact they were many thousands of miles away from home. Often, they were also on their own without the support of loved ones as family members had had to travel on ahead.

As well as providing a listening ear, it was also fascinating to hear people's stories as some of them led such interesting lives and had such colourful tales to tell. Alice and I had hit it off straight away as she was months away from qualifying as a vet and animals have always been a big part of my life. I was enthralled by her 'James Herriot' style tales of her placements on farms and experiences working with horses at the animal hospital. Another patient I brought home once was a retired sea captain and his stories were predictably hilarious, despite being a little rude at times. Definitely one of the most enjoyable aspects of my job was meeting some wonderful people and having time to listen to them – something that is rarely possible in a hospital. Inevitably, there were also some characters that were a real challenge to talk to and the flight couldn't end quickly enough. But they were definitely a minority, and you can't have it all!

Alice went on to make a full recovery and two weeks later the office forwarded a beautiful card that she had made to thank me. She went on to qualify as a vet and a couple of years later made it to the top of the world with a successful Everest summit. A very courageous lady indeed.

CHAPTER 4

Down Time

Back home in between trips I lived with my parents and enjoyed spending time with them. Over the years our relationship had deepened and we had become closer as a family unit, comfortable in each other's company but happy to have our own individual interests as well. The arrangement suited both my parents and me. They gave me a secure anchor point in my otherwise rather nomadic lifestyle whilst I gave them the brightness of youth and the pleasure of sharing in my adventures. Practically, it worked well too. The bills were shared along with the upkeep of the house so finances were less burdensome, and there was no worry about leaving the house empty whilst I was away travelling. My job also meant Mum and Dad had private time together so I never felt as if I was intruding on them.

Of course there were times when we clashed over something and tempers would flare but those incidents were few and far between; generally we got on very well and I regarded them as friends as well as parents. It also benefited me in one other very important way: I never came home to an empty fridge and nothing for tea! Quite the opposite in fact for not only was there always a hot meal waiting for me when I arrived back, but there was often other little treats in store. For example, I once came home from a trip to the States to find that they had redecorated my room for me complete with new carpet, curtains and bedding. They must have worked at some speed as I had only been away four days. But it was such a lovely gesture that I very much appreciated.

Although I would often be away for large chunks of time, I did also get periods where I had a few days off together. This was often much needed as all the travelling could be exhausting, but it also provided time to do things with Mum and Dad. Wrapped up in the busyness of work and socialising with friends, it is so easy to take loved ones for granted and to forget that they are getting older and won't always be there.

Days out to Chester Zoo were a favourite treat with lunch in the café and flasks of coffee to warm us. There were long walks and picnics at our local nature reserve along with movie nights and chocolate-fuelled games of Scrabble where we always invented lots of our own new words (in other words, we cheated!). Such simple little things but they brought so much pleasure.

And a passion for animals - dogs in particular - brightened all our lives. Mum's policy was always 'the more the merrier' so we also had a happy, if somewhat chaotic, house full of boxers and shit tzus. I think at one point we had ten dogs so coming home from a trip was always a boisterous affair involving lots of dog hair and slobber!

When the furore died down Dad would listen avidly to what I'd been up to. Patient confidentiality was always paramount but working around that I would tell him in general terms of the fascinating characters I had met and the crazy, hair-raising moments that I'd had to deal with. (I left out the back alley incident from Kathmandu as I didn't want him to worry.)

Some short, straight forward jobs to France, Spain, Ireland came up, but most of the time it was long haul travelling. I woke up on more than one occasion in a hotel room with no idea what country I was in or what time zone I was on. I once went to Australia, Canada and Malta over an eight day period and was so discombobulated by travelling forward and backward through time zones. Luckily, jet lag didn't usually affect me too much but it could get interesting when I was writing up my patient notes and couldn't remember what day I was on.

Mum also listened with interest to what I'd been up to. Dad and I would almost invariably end up talking about planes and the flying aspect of my job, whereas it was the wildlife and history of the places I visited that drew Mum in. Archaeology captivated her. Shelves of books on Egypt and The Pyramids, Africa and The Great Rift Valley, South America and The Mayan culture lined our living room. When I was able to, I would bring her back a small souvenir from the places I visited; nothing expensive but not the usual cheap and tacky fare a lot of places sell. I took great care choosing and tried to go for authentic bits and pieces crafted by local people. Her favourites were the carved elephant I brought back from Kathmandu and a small wooden boomerang I had made for her by an elderly aboriginal man in the Outback in Australia.

Whilst Dad had undoubtedly sparked the flame of travelling, adventure and flying in me, Mum gave me something else entirely. From her I learned to have a deep understanding and love of caring for people. I learned the true meaning of the word 'family' and what it meant to love unconditionally. And I learned that although kindness and love can't always save people, it can always bring comfort and ease suffering.

All those years ago I had watched her care for Andrea.

Standing outside her room door one morning at the hospital, Dad and I had listened to the sound of Mum's voice softly singing Twinkle Twinkle Little Star. We watched her gently brush Andrea's hair with a blue baby brush then tie a ribbon around her blonde curls to keep them off her face. Next she massaged Andrea's arms and legs with baby lotion, her hands moving slowly and carefully over Andrea's swollen and sore skin, handling each limb as if it were so fragile it could shatter at any moment.

Andrea loved pink, as most little girls do, so whilst she slept, Mum crocheted her a blanket that was soft in its pinkness but warmed her when the chills set in and made her shiver. We watched her tuck this around Andrea, snuggling it up to her chin, all the while continuing to sing softly to her. We stood at the door for ages, Dad and I, not wanting to disturb the moment. Marvelling at how loving and selfless Mum was. I don't know how she did it, day in and day out for six whole months. She was an inspiration. And incredibly brave.

"It's the little things done with love that matter," she said to me later.

As the years passed I then watched her care for Nanna as old age and frailty shrunk her into a shadow of her former self. Patience and love were always plentiful, with time taken to help Nanna knit or make a cake. Baking had always been Nanna's forte and in her younger days she would rustle up delicious pies and scones, crumbles and singing lilies. Knitting and crocheting were also passions; they produced an overflowing wardrobe full of lacy jumpers and beautiful cardigans and dresses that she had made herself, all standing ready for a cruise that she would never go on.

But when illness and confusion swamped her mind, she could no longer remember what to do. Mum would take her to our local market every Friday to buy pretty, pastel-coloured wool. Hours would go by as she sat helping Nanna to make baby clothes. Often, they were not quite right, a few slipped stitches or an uneven hem, but Nanna's eyes would shine with pleasure as she finished her latest creation.

It's something I have carried with me throughout my nursing career both In-Flight and in hospital; something that makes a huge difference to someone's wellbeing. Find out the little things that matter to that person and do them with love. They are often tiny things that are insignificant to others, but to that particular person they mean a lot.

Bringing a lady home from Spain once, she was upset because she'd been taken ill and hadn't been able to get a present for her granddaughter's seventh birthday. After we landed, I asked the driver of our road ambulance to call at the motorway services. The stretcher attracted a few funny looks in WH Smith but she chose a present and a card and was absolutely delighted. Another lady was upset because her hair was a mess and she wanted to look nice for when we landed at Heathrow as her husband was meeting us. A trip into a shop at the airport before we left provided a comb and some lipstick so we were able to make her feel better.

I am very grateful to Mum for being such a wonderful a role model. She led by example, showing me how to love and how to care. The values she gifted me have given me my career and made me a better person. Of course, like most people, I have experienced difficult and sad times but love and kindness have been the things that got me through.

And I have a huge amount of gratitude that I got to spend so much time with my parents, something that not everyone gets the privilege to do.

CHAPTER 5

Italy

The repatriation company employed me on a freelance basis and as such there was always the option to say no to a job. In practise though, I never did. The places I was sent were as varied as they were interesting – some of them so obscure I'd never even heard of them. Many of the calls, as already mentioned, were quite last minute, but usually at sensible times during the day. If a patient was well enough to fly home then they were well enough to wait for their travel to be arranged during normal office hours.

However, one day the phone rang at ten o'clock at night. They wanted me to go with our doctor, Tom, and the air ambulance over to Florence in Italy to collect a 64-year-old lady named Mavis who had had a major stroke whilst on holiday. Exhaustion was weighing me down after a hectic day and the temptation to say no was swirling around alongside images of my bed and a good long sleep. But when I heard the words 'air ambulance' the tiredness shape shifted into a jolt of excitement. It would be my first time on the air ambulance; the real cutting edge of the job. I had been waiting and hoping for this very moment so wasn't about to miss it.

We were to leave at 6am the following morning from the air ambulance base at an airfield in Oxford. I would have to grab a couple of hours sleep and then leave at 2am to meet Tom and the flight team. Although I *was* very tired, it would not be an insurmountable problem –working through the night was something I had done many times, often surviving on very little sleep, so

I knew I could dig deep and the energy would be there when needed. And, of course, excitement produces lots of adrenaline which is like having rocket fuel coursing through your veins.

There was one small issue. I had just picked up a new car, literally just a few hours earlier, and had no petrol. I had planned to fill up in the morning. Not being used to filling up at night I wracked my brains trying to think where there might be an open garage. And then I remembered that I had seen one that was open 24 hours a day when coming back from a trip one night; it wasn't far away on the busy dual carriageway near where I live. Sorted, I thought, I will just call in on my way and then jump on the motorway. I duly headed off to bed.

Predictably, sleep danced around but eluded me when I tried to catch it. My brain told me it was far too risky to nod off in case I slept through my 1.30am wake up call. So I gave up trying and crept quietly down stairs, trying not to wake the whole household in the process, and made myself a cup of steaming coffee to savour before I left. The gentle snoring of the dogs thrummed in the background as they slept and was the only sound in the early morning stillness. They hadn't stirred, content and safe and completely unperturbed by me creeping around.

As I sat sipping my drink, the muted light from the cooker display cast a soft blue glow over the kitchen, and I realised I felt content and safe too. Our home with its warm kitchen and pile of sleeping dogs was my safe place, the place that enabled me to confidently head out into the dark knowing I had my anchor point to return to. I took a few moments to do some deep breathing exercises to relax me before this latest adventure began. Not really knowing what to expect, the one thing I did know was that the day would undoubtedly be pretty full on.

The front door clicked softly behind me as the house ushered me out into the night. A couple of minutes later the small issue of needing fuel morphed into a bit of a problem. Standing at a petrol pump on a deserted garage forecourt at two o'clock in the morning, my petrol locking cap was stuck tight. I couldn't budge it. It was the first time I'd filled up the new car but as I'd been driving for many years had never even given it a thought other than where would be open. My key slid in, the lock turned, but the cap didn't. I tried and tried but was frightened of breaking the key so couldn't use too much brute force. I looked around and an utterly deserted forecourt stared back at me. I headed to the window to ask the cashier for help but he politely told me he was locked in for his own safety and wasn't allowed to come out. What was I going to do? Normally, as I guess lots of young people would do, if I had a problem like this I would just call my Dad and he would ride to my rescue, twiddle something or other and fix it - often with a can of WD40 somewhere in the mix. But it was two o'clock in the morning. Definitely not an option this time.

Returning to my car, I tried again. Eventually, after twenty minutes of struggling, and out of sheer desperation, I gave it an almighty thump with my tyre iron and miraculously it freed it. Relief flooded over me. The air ambulance would be waiting for me and if I hadn't shown up it could have meant the whole trip being cancelled. This would have been devastating for Mavis and her family and potentially very expensive for my company as I didn't know what fees etc. they would have to pay. It would also have been massively embarrassing for me to explain the reason why I hadn't shown up on time and could have had consequences for my continued employment with them. In short, it could have been a disaster. But it wasn't, thank goodness, so I took a deep breath to steady myself and climbed in the car to get going. Now running late, I had to get a move on. Luckily, the traffic angels were looking out for me that night and the motorway was clear. I made good time and even arrived at the airfield in Oxford with a few minutes to spare.

But as I pulled up, the airfield was a blanket of inky blackness and looked deserted. There didn't appear to be anyone about at all. My headlights found a large sign by the side of the gates that told me I was definitely in the right place so I drove around a couple of times trying to figure out how to get in. And then out of the darkness came another set of headlights swinging into the car park. It was Tom, the doctor I would be traveling with.

Tom was also the founder and owner of the repatriation company so I was a little nervous. I hoped my newbie nerves wouldn't make me fumble about too much and that I wouldn't embarrass myself with any major gaffs. I had done my In-Flight training course with Tom prior to starting work so although this was the first time I would be working with him I had met him and spent a little time with him. A confident but pleasant man, he seemed easy going as well as supremely knowledgeable. Many years as a trauma specialist in the army had led him to set up his own company and it appeared that there was little, if anything, that he didn't know about aviation medicine. At a slim five feet seven with close cropped sandy hair and serious brown eyes, he wasn't physically imposing, but he had a way about him that instantly put you at ease and made you feel as if you were in good hands. A much-valued trait in a doctor, the so-called 'bedside manner' is a powerful asset. Surprisingly, over the years, I met very few medics who actually had this magic ingredient; it's a quality inherent to a person's make up rather than something that can be taught, and arguably, it's of equal importance to clinical skill. From my perspective, being able to relate to and trust who you are working with makes for a much better working atmosphere; being able to rely on their judgement and know they will listen and work with you rather than just steam-roller on. Something that is often said in healthcare settings is that you can cope with anything if you have the right team around you. Although I suppose this is true of any profession not just healthcare. So, on seeing Tom, I relaxed a little, sensing that working with him would be a pleasure. And this is my chance, I thought, to learn everything I can about working on the air ambulance.

Tom produced a set of keys that opened the gate and allowed us access to the airfield. A small portakabin loomed up ahead in the darkness and in it we found our two pilots pouring over their charts and planning our route. Introductions were made, coffee rustled up and then we had a short briefing. Tom was also a qualified pilot so there were a few minutes of aviation technical talk and then we moved onto our patient.

It seemed Mavis had had a large haemorrhagic stroke, or bleed, at the base of her brain, an area known as the brain stem. This structure governs the major functions of the body, including respiration, so an event like this can be catastrophic and often immediately fatal. Against the odds, she had survived the initial period but was very poorly. There was a real chance she might not recover so her family wanted her brought home to the UK as soon as possible so that she could be cared for in a local hospital with her family all nearby. The plan was to do the trip in one day: fly out early, meet the road ambulance on the apron at the airport in Italy, load Mavis on board and then fly back to Oxford. We would then be met by another road ambulance that would transport Mavis to a local hospital where a bed had been arranged for her.

Everything was looking good weather-wise so when Tom had finished the briefing we headed out into the chilly morning air. The fixed-wing air ambulance sat a hundred metres in front of us shrouded in an ethereal cloud of mist that hung over the air-field. I could just make out the wings and the fuselage. I knew the plane wouldn't be very big but I was a little surprised to see just how small it actually was. Inside there was two seats up front for the pilots. In the back, a stretcher was anchored along the side of the aircraft facing the door while two seats, one behind the other, sat on the opposite side. And that was it. We had with us a small heart monitor, a portable suction machine in case we needed to clear Mavis's airway, a red emergency bag full of drugs and intubation equipment for if we needed to take over Mavis's breathing for her, and a portable ventilator. On top of that, we had our small personal bags with us, so by the time everything was stowed away on board it was pretty snug.

Tom and I got ourselves settled, the pilots did their pre-flight checks, and then we started rolling out towards the runway. I suppressed my mounting excitement and maintained my professional demeanour but inside I was having one of those 'pinch me' moments – I couldn't believe I was actually here doing this. Every nerve in my body was fizzing with the thrill of it. The runway lights flashed into view through the lingering mist and we were cleared for take-off. It was a little bumpier than I was used to but as the wheels cleared the ground and we headed into the newly dawning sky it was other worldly. Take off is always my favourite part of flying and this one didn't disappoint. The roar of the engines, the giddy sensation as you leave the ground, the knowledge that you are free of the Earth and heading into the great blue yonder - just captivating. No matter how many times I did it, it never lost its thrill factor. And as the cliché goes, I would have done this job for nothing. It was just an added bonus that I was being paid too.

We knew it would be pretty full on once we picked Mavis up so Tom and I used the time on the outbound journey to check all our equipment, read all the case notes so we were fully up to speed on all Mavis's previous medical history, and agree our care plan. We also knew that opportunities to eat and drink would be limited once we had Mavis on board so we ate sandwiches and drank more coffee that the pilots had thoughtfully provided for us so that we were set up for the day ahead. I had naively thought there would be a toilet on board but quickly realised there wasn't so did have to go easy on the coffee!

The flight was smooth and uneventful and we landed as scheduled at the airport in Italy. We weren't actually going to enter the country through immigration, but were meeting the ambulance airside, loading Mavis on board and then leaving again. It literally was just a land, load and leave. The pilots taxied us around as instructed by air traffic control and sure enough the ambulance with Mavis on board was parked up and waiting for us at the designated meeting point.

As we disembarked, the paramedics wasted to time. The ambulance doors were already open and they were unloading the stretcher with Mavis strapped to it, a red blanket wrapped tightly around her and an oxygen mask over her face. As Tom and I walked towards them, we instantly saw why. The brief had been that Mavis was 'poorly' but she was clearly 'exceedingly' poorly. Her face was the colour of putty and her breathing was laboured and intermittent – a type of breathing known as 'Cheyne Stoking' whereby the patient has long periods in between breaths where it can appear as if they have actually died. In fact, it is usually the type of breathing that does precede death. Tom caught my eye and I nodded to acknowledge that I was thinking the same thing he was: would Mavis actually survive the flight home? We had to balance the indignity of her dying on board the flight, and the legal implications of a death in international airspace, with the compassionate and caring desire to get her back to her family so she could die at home. We knew if we didn't take her now she definitely wouldn't get a second chance. All her family had gone on ahead and she would die alone in a foreign hospital. But we also knew she might not make it. Would she be able to hang on long enough to get home?

After a brief moment of consideration, Tom made the decision to accept her and to try. In that instant I was very relieved to be travelling with him and to not be responsible for having to make that call myself. It was the case sometimes that the decisions we had to make whilst on a job had huge implications both from a medical point of view and a financial one. For example, the pilot of a commercial airliner would divert and make an emergency landing if we felt it was medically necessary, but the cost to the airline was enormous, and there was the inconvenience to all the other passengers to consider. Tom had told us on the training course that we were the ones actually at the scene and that whatever we decided was necessary he and the company would back us one hundred percent. But - and there is always a 'but', isn't there? - he stressed that we must be absolutely certain in our minds that such drastic action was needed and that we had the clinical data to back up our decision. It was a huge responsibility not to be taken lightly so on this occasion I was happy to hand the decision over to him.

Decision made, we set about loading Mavis into the air ambulance. There plane was equipped with a special mechanism, a kind of mechanical arm, that made manoeuvring the stretcher on board easier so we quickly got her transferred over and fastened in ready for take-off. I wired her up to our heart and oxygen monitors. Her oxygen levels were predictably low and the screen of the heart monitor displayed a heart rate that jumped about erratically. When I attached the blood pressure cuff to her arm, her blood pressure was so low it was difficult to record. The truth of the matter was that Mavis had begun the dying process and her body was slowly and steadily shutting down. I wrapped her up warmly in several more blankets and propped her up in a semi upright position to aid her breathing and make her as comfortable as possible. She was still conscious at this point, although it was doubtful if she actually knew what was happening. After we had done everything needed and were seated ready for take-off, I reached over to hold Mavis's hand. Talking quietly to her, I told her our names and explained what was going to happen next. I chatted on about her grandchildren – her case notes said she had three - and although she was so poorly, she squeezed my hand and managed the smallest of smiles. My heart ached for her having to go through all of this, and at only sixty-four-years of age. A very similar age in fact to my Mum and Dad at that time. I hoped if it ever came to it that someone would look after them with kindness and compassion. I resolved to make Mavis's journey home as comfortable and dignified as possible.

We were part way into the flight when Mavis started to deteriorate rapidly. Already in a serious condition it didn't take much before her condition became critical. She stopped responding at all to us and her blood pressure fell so low it was un-recordable. Glancing at the pulse oximeter I saw her oxygen levels plummet despite her being on 100% oxygen via a face mask. The heart monitor displayed a see-saw of erratic, chaotic beats interspersed with long and troubling pauses. Already on an intravenous drip, Tom turned it on full and I whipped open the emergency bag and readied drugs and intubation equipment.

And then she started to vomit. Great gushing spurts of brown fluid. I grabbed the portable suction machine we had brought with us and attached a plastic yanker – a rigid suction tube – to the end of the pipe and began to suck her mouth out in an effort to stop her choking. In that moment it became glaringly obvious how difficult it is to manage a vomiting, unconscious patient in such a confined space. Quickly dropping the head of the stretcher flat, Tom extended Mavis's neck to open up her airway whilst I continued using the yanker to suck up the vomit which just kept coming and coming. The portable machine was doing its best, but it was a losing battle. Vomit soaked into the sheets and splattered onto the floor and side of the aircraft. In such a confined space the smell was terrible. Even though vomit was nothing new to us, its sour smell threatened to make us both gag.

Tom was staring intently at Mavis.

"What do you want to do?" I asked.

"We need to intubate," he said. "And land."

I nodded and reached for the ET tube that he would insert into Mavis's trachea. He turned to alert the pilots.

By this time we were flying over France. The pilots put out an emergency call and we were granted permission to make an emergency landing on the airstrip of a nearby French military airbase. Tom swiftly intubated Mavis as we started our decent through the clouds. She was still making some respiratory effort herself but the tube going down into her lungs would protect her airway and stop her aspirating the foul brown vomit. It also enabled us to deliver oxygen more efficiently. Within minutes, we had landed and were taxiing towards a group of fire engines and soldiers that had hastily been scrambled to meet us.

Mavis continued to vomit intermittently but thankfully it was now just a few millilitres each time rather than the voluminous amounts she had been producing. However, her breathing had become even more laboured so Tom was now helping her breath with the Ambu bag connected to the end of the endotracheal tube he had inserted. The suction machine still rattled away when needed and I was attempting to clean her up a little before we moved her. Touching her skin, her hands were ice blocks. Luckily there were a couple of spare blankets tucked away under the seats so I quickly wrapped her up ever more tightly in an effort to warm her. Her temperature was unrecordable.

The aircraft rolled to a stop and the door was immediately flung open. I found myself face-to-face with a soldier dressed head to toe in black combat clothing. A balaclava hid his face except for his eyes which lasered into me with a stare so hard it made the hairs on the back of my neck stand on end. He held a machine gun in front of him, his finger by the trigger. He didn't speak, just held my gaze for many more seconds than was comfortable. On the tarmac outside were another five or six soldiers standing shoulder to shoulder in a solid black line. They all brandished the same machine guns. I glanced nervously at Tom. He seemed completely unfazed and continued to squeeze air into Mavis's lungs as if he faced soldiers with machine guns every day. I guess with having been in the army maybe he had done on many occasions. His calm manner reassured me a little but it was still very intimidating.

Obviously, with it being a military airbase, security was a major concern, but after a few more seconds of scrutinising the cabin, the lead man seemed satisfied that it was a genuine medical emergency. He lowered his gun and signalled the all clear to his fellow soldiers. They slung their guns over their shoulders and pitched in to get the stretcher off the aircraft. I busied myself collecting the equipment we would need to take with us, but couldn't stop my eyes drifting over to those machine guns every now and then.

One of the waiting vehicles, a red fire engine/ambulance, drove forward and Mavis was loaded into the back. There was three staff on board the vehicle that looked like they were paramedics. Quickly and efficiently they secured the stretcher in place and hooked Mavis up to their oxygen supply as ours was running low.

Two of the paramedics climbed in up front and, with no warning, they suddenly took off at breakneck speed, screeching across the airfield with all the lights and sirens going. Tom and I

DID I PACK MY STETHOSCOPE?

were thrown backwards and just managed to grab onto the side of the vehicle to stop ourselves ending up on the floor. It was a long five-minute journey and extremely challenging continuing to care for Mavis whilst being flung around the back of the vehicle at seventy plus miles per hour.

And then it suddenly dawned on me that in all the rush I had forgotten to grab my rucksack. It was still on board the air ambulance. I was now racing to a hospital in France with no passport, no money, no anything. It was another rookie mistake and I cursed myself. Yet another valuable lesson was learned: always keep your bag glued to you.

The blazing ambulance delivered us to a sprawling, old-fashioned looking hospital. I was glad the journey wasn't a long one as bruises were already blooming on my arms from being tossed about like flotsam in the back of the vehicle.

A team of staff in blue scrubs were waiting for us; they ran us through the emergency department into a spacious cubicle lined with monitors and equipment. Around us, the usual beeps and alarms of a busy resus area echoed off the walls along with a ringing phone and the hum of voices. We all pitched in and transferred Mavis smoothly over to the waiting trolley and then the doctor in charge called for quiet. Tom quickly and concisely handed over to them what had happened – his French fluid and assured.

The decision was immediately made to put Mavis onto a ventilator to breath for her. If I'm honest I was rather dismayed to hear this. Mavis was in the middle of the dying process so I found it upsetting that she should have to be put through this. In my opinion it would have been far kinder to make her comfortable and just sit with her as she passed away. In her current state, without the ventilator to breath for her, it wouldn't have taken long. I understood why they were doing it: she had collapsed whilst in transit so they wanted to give her a chance. And there was also her family to consider. Putting her on a ventilator would buy time for them to get to their Mum's side so they could be with her. And all these considerations had to be weighed up in a matter of seconds so in view of that I suppose it was a sensible decision. But I still felt a hollow sense of sadness for Mavis. It's always been my belief that providing a peaceful, dignified death when the outcome is inevitable is just as important as fighting tooth and nail to save someone who has a chance. Unfortunately, it's not always clear cut; there is always the grey area in between.

The team quickly got to work and Mavis was put on a ventilator with the minimum of fuss. As the machine took over breathing for Mavis and she stabilised, the cubicle emptied of staff apart from one nurse who busied herself filling in paperwork. Spying my chance, I moved over to give Mavis's hand a squeeze and have a moment with her before heading outside through the heaving reception area to the front of the hospital. I would wait with our equipment whilst Tom accompanied Mavis to the Intensive Care Unit.

Across the road from the A&E, a small patch of grass with a couple of trees and a bench provided a quiet corner so I gratefully headed over and sat down. It had been a full on day; not entirely unexpected but non-the-less challenging and thought provoking, with a few twists and turns I hadn't anticipated. Taking a few deep breaths had become my go-to method for relaxing so I inhaled slowly to the count of four then out again to the count of four. Closing my eyes momentarily, the sun warmed my face and I felt my pulse rate start to slow. The effects of having so little sleep the night before were beginning to surface; tiredness was racing up behind me along with the inevitable crash from the adrenaline high that the emergency had produced. But I knew I had to keep going as the day was not over yet so I allowed myself a few more moments of deep breathing, attempting to still my mind and metaphorically regroup. I didn't quite manage it but I did feel better.

As I hadn't got my bag, and therefore no money either, I couldn't buy a drink so decided to sort out our equipment and then see if the staff on reception in A&E would let me have a glass of water as I was also developing a headache from dehydration. With monitors, our emergency bag and the mattress from our stretcher to look after, there was a lot of equipment so moving around much was impossible. The heart monitor was very expensive – around ten thousand pounds at the time – and the emergency bag was full of drugs and needles/syringes so I couldn't let them out of my sight.

Across the road the hospital was in full flow with staff, patients and relatives buzzing around and ambulances pulling in every few minutes. A member of staff who looked like a porter strolled out of the building and headed in my direction. I decided to be cheeky and ask if he knew where I could get some water. Luckily, he spoke English as my French is non-existent, and after I explained what had happened he very kindly went and got me a couple of bottles of water from their staff room.

The light slowly lowered around me as it got later and later. With no other option, I had to just sit and patiently wait. Coldness was creeping around me too and I was debating on gathering the equipment up and going in search of somewhere warmer when Tom stepped out of the doors looking tired and drained. I waved and he headed over towards me. He carried his professional demeanour well, but I could see the sadness in his eyes and guessed that he too had been troubled by the decisions that had had to be taken today.

"She's ventilated and stable at the moment," he said, as he sat down beside me. "But we need to contact her family immediately."

I nodded.

"And we have another little problem," he went on. "The airfield in Oxford closes at 11pm - I don't know if we'll make it back in time so the plane might have to go without us."

My heart dropped like a brick. My bag was on the plane.

Tom gratefully accepted the bottle of water I had saved for him and then headed back into the hospital to make some calls and see what could be organised.

Great, I thought to myself. We're going to have to stay over in a hotel and I have nothing at all with me, not even a jumper to protect against the evening chill. Then the fact I had no passport crashed through my mind like a Stormtrooper and anger started to bubble up. How could I have been so stupid to put myself in this position? I would also have to tell Tom. I suddenly felt very tired and very foolish.

But then we had a stroke of luck. Tom headed back out saying that he had contacted Mavis's daughter and she would be flying straight out with her brother. And he had managed to call in a favour. They were going to keep the airfield in Oxford open for us so the air ambulance could wait and we could all head back home together that night. We had also been fortunate in that when Tom spoke to our pilots they were able to arrange a military car to come and pick us up.

Back at the air base, the air ambulance was refuelled and ready to go. Clambering wearily back on board, Tom and I cleaned our equipment the best we could with antibacterial wipes and stowed it all away whilst the pilots waited for clearance to leave. The smell of vomit still lingered, and everything would need to be deep cleaned, but we had got rid of the worst of it.

The excitement of the morning seemed as if it had happened twenty years ago, and it had been replaced by a grubby exhaustion that spoke volumes about the reality of life as an In-Flight nurse. Hours without the opportunity for a toilet break or freshen up; no food or drink all day except one bottle of water; equipment covered in vomit that had to be cleaned. It was a far cry from the glamorous job my friends all kidded me about, thinking I spent all day chatting away to handsome pilots and having five course meals on the expense account.

Jim, the older of our two pilots, had managed to get us a flask of hot coffee and a Twix each. Both Tom and I were absolutely starving so it was the best chocolate bar I'd ever eaten and we both devoured the coffee in a matter of minutes. Jim settled back up front and the glowing lights of the runway beckoned us on into the darkness. Soon, we were airborne and on our way home.

The atmosphere in the cabin was quiet and sombre. I couldn't shake off the feeling that we had failed Mavis. We had so wanted to get her home to her family. But it wasn't meant to be. I couldn't help thinking of her poor son and daughter now racing to get to their Mum's side. What a horrible situation for them to find themselves in. Tom seemed to sense what I was thinking, or maybe he was thinking the same thing, for he suddenly turned to me and said simply,

"We tried."

I nodded. "Yes, we did. And for what it's worth I think you made a good call."

And then on impulse I blurted out, "I made a stupid mistake."

Tom raised his eyebrows and looked questioningly at me.

"I left my bag on the plane. I had no passport or money with me. If the plane had left without us it would have caused loads of hassle."

I didn't need to have said anything, I had 'got away' with it, but it was weighing heavily on me so I instantly felt better for having told him.

He smiled wryly at me in the glowing lights from the cockpit. "If I had a pound for every time I'd done that I would be a rich man."

"Seriously?"

"Seriously," he replied.

I nodded. "Thank you."

"No problem."

A blaze of lights welcomed us back to the runway in Oxford. It was 11.30pm. We taxied back to the hanger. A ghostly eeriness dropped on us when we disembarked as the runway lights suddenly clicked off and total blackness enveloped the airfield.

Tom decided we all needed food and a little boost so offered to buy us all supper. It was very late but Jim knew an Indian restaurant that would still be open so we all piled into Tom's car and headed off. He treated us to a delicious meal which we all fell on like hyenas on a fresh carcass. The guys were great company, and as all three of them were pilots, the talk was mostly about aviation so right up my street. It was great to forget about the stresses of the day and just relax and it did occur to me that I was now chatting with handsome pilots and enjoying a five star meal on the expense account. But after we had eaten I could no longer keep my eyes open and was too tired to really care about anything other than sleep. It was now 1am and I had been on the go since 2am the previous morning.

Now came the challenge of finding a hotel in the middle of the night as driving back to Manchester was definitely out of the question at this point. Jim came to the rescue again and directed us to a local Holiday Inn. We called ahead to check they had a room and then Tom dropped me at the door – along with my precious bag! I would collect my car from the airfield and drive home the next day.

I was exhausted and grubby so settled into bed with a deep sigh and no small measure of relief. But sleep once again eluded me. In some ways I felt a sense of satisfaction. I had ticked off my first air ambulance repatriation, keeping calm whilst on a French military air base surrounded by soldiers with guns. And watching Tom calmly orchestrate the events of the day had been a masterclass on how to handle such a scenario. But, although I had kept my head and worked steadily, the thought that I had been just a 'hanger on' whilst Tom did what was needed was taunting me like the meanest of school bullies. A shrill and insistent voice at the back of my head telling me I was massively out of my depth. 'You do know Tom could have done the job without you, don't you? You couldn't even manage to remember to take your bag with you!' And then lower and more menacing: 'And what about Frank? Without Dan you would have lost him. And Kathmandu where you could have got yourself murdered?' Tiredness was no doubt making things worse but the thought that I wasn't good enough to do this job was beginning to take shape in a very real way.

Two days later Tom rang me to say that Mavis had passed away at the hospital in France. But her son and daughter had made it to her side and she had been comfortable and pain free. Rest easy, beautiful lady, it was an honour to look after you.

CHAPTER 6

Growing Up 1969-1980

Thick fog shrouds much of my childhood after Andrea died. I remember very little, almost as if by blocking everything out my six-year-old brain was trying to protect itself. I don't remember her funeral or going back to school; I don't remember that first Christmas without her; I don't remember going on days out or doing things, although I'm sure we must have. Only snippets of images are there, indistinct and blurry, and no amount of trying to focus in on them makes them any clearer. But one thing that is front and centre, clear and sharp in my memory, is the need I felt to care for and protect my Mum.

My parents had already lost their first child, Paul, when he was eighteen months old – two years before I was born and eight years before Andrea died – so the loss of another child was too much for Mum to bear. She sank into a deep and all-consuming depression, more or less ceasing to function in any meaningful way. I remember her sitting by the coal fire staring into the flames for hours at a time, not speaking or engaging with us in any way. She would forget to eat or drink and all the things she loved to do were sucked away by the black vacuum of grief. Her world became meaningless.

Every day before school I would comb her hair and hold her hand for a little while; I never wanted to leave her.

Dad got a job in an electrical wiring factory and worked hard to support us and try to get some money together whilst Nanna looked after Mum and me. Although by no means ideal – as already mentioned we were all cramped together in Nanna's two bedroom terraced house – I suppose it was probably a good thing as Mum was completely unable to look after herself or us. Mental health care at that time was very poor, and bereavement counselling non-existent, so Mum was just left to suffer. Even though I was so young, I saw her sadness for the very real thing it was, and although not properly able to understand it, I empathized deeply with her and 'got it'. I had my own grief wrapped around me as I had lost my best friend who I did everything with so I didn't need to understand it, I just instinctively felt where she was coming from. My main purpose in life became trying to care for her and cheer her up. I desperately wanted her to be happy again because I suppose, as children do, I equated Mum being happy with everything being ok again. Although in reality things were never going to be 'ok again' in the same sense as they had been before.

For many weeks I saved my pocket money and one day took myself off to the local Co Op up the road. It was not a supermarket like it is now but a homewares and gift shop. I wanted to get Mum something to make her smile. It was much safer then than now so I happily trotted off on my own – I think I must have been about seven at the time. After wandering around for a while, I saw, and fell in love with, a bright purple orchid flower arrangement in a pretty pearly white pot that sparkled in the light. The flowers were artificial but were so vibrant and colourful I thought it would be perfect. I didn't look at the price ticket and didn't have any concept of what things cost, so I just carefully picked up the flowers and made my way to the till. I had five pounds in my purse which at the time seemed like an enormous amount of money. Of course, it was nowhere near enough.

"It's to cheer my Mum up," I told the lady at the till. "She's not been well after my sister died."

The lady smiled at me with kind blue eyes and gently explained that I didn't have enough money and that I would have to go and ask my Dad for some more if I wanted to buy it. Disappointment threatened to produce tears. I knew Dad would have no spare money to give me so I left the shop without the flowers, feeling totally dejected. Little did I know, or grasp the concept, that flowers, no matter how beautiful, would not make my Mum smile again. It would be like trying to build a house with drawing pins.

Dad never talked about or showed his feelings. I guess men, particularly of his generation, often didn't. He just worked hard and did his best to hold things together.

Another thing I do remember vividly is sitting at the kitchen table with him in the evenings watching him draw pictures of the planes he had worked with in the RAF. As his pencil sketched across the paper, he would tell me stories to make me laugh about how he used to wear ladies tights under his uniform to keep warm when working on the airfields at night during the bitter German winters. And about how he unwittingly caused a major incident one day by leaving a bag of laundry outside the NAAFI shop in Laarbruch sparking a bomb scare. The more evenings we sat together the more elaborate his stories became. His words carried me away to foreign lands were there were camels and rhino, and elephants and tigers. We visited the floating markets in Thailand and the Golden Pagoda in China. Accompanying us was a whole cast of colourful characters. He started doing funny voices and drawing cartoons to illustrate his tales and I would sit for hours hanging on to his every word. I became enthralled with the idea of flying, exploring and seeking out new adventures.

Looking back now I can see how this not only benefited me but would have helped him enormously too. His struggle must have been every bit as hard as Mum's as he had not only lost two children but had also had to give up the RAF career he loved. His dreams of travelling the world and working with planes had been ripped out from under him. On top of that he had lost his home, and the woman he loved had become little more than a shell of her former self. He must have fought valiantly to keep his own despair at bay. And his stories and beautiful drawings were his weapons of choice.

Many times Dad would try to pull Mum into the adventure

with us but she would just continue to stare into the fire or go up to bed.

Throughout this time Nanna quietly went about the business of doing her best to care for us all. Money was scarce but baking was something she excelled at so there were always the comforting aromas of meat and potato pies in the oven and apple crumbles made from cheap apples picked up on the market. My favourite was her 'singing lilies' – flat pastry pockets full of currants – that we would slather with butter and eat warm from the oven. For a real treat she would bake a loaf of crusty white bread and slice off great chunks that we would then skewer with a knife and toast over the open fire.

Prior to writing this book, images of old age wrinkling Nanna's face and driving her into dementia were all I could summon up. To my shame I recall being scared of her as she sat talking to herself and ripping pieces of paper up into hundreds of tiny bits. Her illness and confusion wiped everything else out. But focusing on this time in order to write about it brought forth images of her before this happened. It enabled me to remember her baking for us and looking after us when Mum couldn't. There was always a roaring fire warming the house and clean clothes carefully mended and ironed ready for school. I found I could even recall tiny details like the red slippers she wore and the pink frilly apron that protected her from flour as she worked. She was so much more than the illness and old age that consumed her and I will be forever grateful for the love and compassion she showered us with when everything else in our world was bleak and empty.

Mum's depression did eventually start to slowly improve but for the rest of her life it lurked around in the shadows and would sometimes come raging out of the corner and knock her off her feet for a few weeks at a time. The desire to care for her and try to make things better always stayed with me. And there was an element of 'survivor's guilt' there too. Why did Andrea die and I didn't? I felt guilty that I had lived, and that somehow I had to make it up to Mum and try and fill the huge hole that Andrea left.

Of course, none of what happened was my fault and I was never going to be able to fill that void no matter what I did. Strangely though, even into adulthood, that feeling never left me. I always felt the need to try and make it up to her.

As Mum slowly emerged from the black hole of depression, she decided to apply to be an Enrolled Nurse. At the time, there were two levels in nursing: State Registered Nurses (SRNs) and State Enrolled Nurses (SENs). The former involved three years of training and the latter two. Leigh Infirmary accepted her on to their two year course. We all hoped that this new focus would help her heal and bring back the smiling young woman that she had once been.

On her first day she came downstairs in her dark green uniform with a pristine, starched white apron and shiny black shoes that Dad had polished for her. She must have been terrified of putting herself out into the world again but her strength shone through and she bravely accepted the challenge. I was so proud of her. And absolutely thrilled when she gave me a big hug and a gentle smile before she left.

For the next few weeks Mum adjusted to the shift patterns and worked hard. Dad whispered his stories at the kitchen table so that we wouldn't disturb her as she studied. Seeing her by the fire with her books spread on her lap busily working away was a tonic for us all, a stark contrast from the previous vacant months. Nanna encouraged her to get her hair done; Dad treated her to a new coat. And then one evening she actually joined us at the kitchen table to listen to one of Dad's stories. It was such a simple thing but its significance to Dad and me felt gargantuan.

Sadly though, a new and completely unexpected development stopped her in her tracks. The stress she had endured from Andrea's death had caused her to develop asthma. At the time nurses used copious amounts of talcum powder when they were caring for patients and Mum couldn't cope with it. An allergy to the talc caused one asthma attack after another and ended her nursing dreams. After three months of persevering she had to admit it wasn't going to work. Fear that this new disappointment would send her spiralling downwards again ate into me, the unfairness of it felt unbearable. For the next few weeks I invented sore throats and headaches so that I could stay home from school and be with her; I thought that I could hold back the blackness and stop it getting to her.

But then, just as bad things can pop up with no warning, so can good things. Something else happened completely unexpectedly that would prove to be a real turning point and would breathe new life into us all . . . literally. Mum found out that she was pregnant.

Three years had gone by since Andrea died. I was nine years old and about to become a big sister again.

My school friends squealed with delight when I eagerly ran into class telling them all the news. Mrs Foley, my softly spoken and kind hearted teacher, allowed us all to spend some of the morning making congratulations cards for Mum. Such a thoughtful gesture that made my day.

On the 2nd of March 1972, Caroline eased her way into our world. She was perfect in every way with Dad's gentle blue eyes and feather-soft wisps of blonde hair curling over her forehead. Our house sprang into life as if a touch paper had been lit and she coloured Mum's face with a glow we hadn't seen for years. Holding Caroline for the first time, I felt an enormous wave of love course through me. I couldn't take my eyes off her. Every detail of her tiny fingers curled around mine captivated me. And when she looked at me the connection was instant; I knew we would be life-long friends and that I would do everything in my power to protect her and care for her. No one would ever hurt her whilst I was there to look out for her.

This is also the point when my memory becomes much clearer again. Caroline's arrival swept away the fog that clouded my mind for so long and I have many distinct memories from this time.

As I was old enough, I helped out with feeds and changing nappies. Hours passed rocking her in her pram, playing with her and singing nursery rhymes. It gave Mum some much needed time to look after herself and I was delighted to be trusted enough to help. It also meant that the close bond we already had deepened very quickly; in short, I adored her.

Then on the 15th May 1974 – Andrea's fifth anniversary – Mum had another baby, a little boy. I'm sure for my parents the bitter sweet element would have been profound but for Caroline and me it was a joyous moment: we had a new baby brother. In Andrea's honour, they named him Andrew.

The sun grinned down that day and everything seemed bluer and brighter and blossomed over with colour. Caroline and I were playing together in the back yard whilst Mum was in labour in the front room. The midwife had arrived at twelve o'clock and I was making sure we played quietly so that we could hear what was going on and didn't miss anything.

Then at 2.15pm Andrew's first cry reached our straining ears. Caroline giggled as I whipped her up and spun her round in excitement. Even the birds swooped lower and faster as if they too were joining in the celebrations. Dad came bounding out of the house to tell us the news and then he ran off to the corner shop to get pop and treats so that we could have a little party. (As a young man Dad ran everywhere, seeming to have a boundless supply of energy.)

A little while later Nanna ushered us in to meet our new baby brother and I was so excited I could hardly contain myself. Andrew also had Dad's blue eyes but the thing I loved the most about him was the gentle upturn of his lips that made him look as if he was smiling at us. At ten pounds in weight, it was amazing Mum had managed a normal delivery – she was only five-feet-one-inch tall and weighed seven stones. But she had, he was healthy, and we now had a new member of our little gang; two had become three.

I'm sure it was coincidence that Andrew was born on Andrea's anniversary but it was a deeply poignant moment for Mum. Although not particularly religious, she told me years later that she definitely felt as if she had been given a gift from God that day. And we all felt our grief-laden hearts lightening a little more.

Helping to look after my baby brother and toddler sister continued to develop the caring, nurturing side of my personality. I loved every minute of my time with them. Dad's kitchen-table story sessions continued only now we each had a little one on our knee and the stories featured dinosaurs and princesses as well as planes and foreign lands.

As I moved into my teenage years, and Caroline and Andrew got older, I started to take them on little adventures. Trips to the park became days out in Blackpool and Southport; we laughed our way through pantomimes and shows; and then eventually train trips to London provided history and excitement.

Thinking back on it with today's glasses on, it was very brave of Mum to let us do the things she did. Initially after Andrea died I had been cossetted and protected, never being allowed to play out in case something happened to me. Learning to ride a bike never happened in case I fell off and hurt myself, and the swimming baths were a no-no as I could have drowned. It inhibited me to a large extent and my social skills definitely developed slower than those of my peers. It was a cotton wool existence spun out of fear and grief. A very understandable reaction after the losses Mum had suffered. So to then allow me as a teenager to take Caroline and Andrew, who were still very young, all the way to London, on my own, must have taken a mountain of courage. I can imagine her sitting there nervously waiting as the clock ticked on. Waiting and wondering and hoping we would return safely. And this was before the time of mobile phones so a quick text or call to check we were ok wasn't an option. But for me, I was in my element, finally spreading my wings and flying free. Many hours were spent wandering around and seeing the sights, eating ice cream in Hyde Park and fighting off the pigeons attempting to steal our sandwiches in Trafalgar Square. How Mum must have yearned to keep the three of us safe and cocooned at home, but the realisation that she couldn't, that she had to let us go out into the world, must have become clearer as her own spirit blossomed back into life. And I guess she probably accepted that she couldn't really stop us anyway, that wanderlust would win out in the end no matter what she did.

By this time my love of exploring and discovering new places was stitched into every strand of my personality. Dad had created an image of an exciting and wondrous world. He had brought to life the colours, the sounds, the scents of all that lay beyond the confines of our kitchen table. Flying off and seeing it for myself was now my ultimate goal.

And my career choice was also now firmly set; there were never really any other contenders, nothing that ever came close to what I wanted to do. I wanted to be a nurse and I wanted to look after people. It was as simple as that.

CHAPTER 7

Antigua

I waited on tenterhooks for a few days after I got back from the air ambulance trip to Italy. Tom hadn't said anything on the day but I wondered if there may be some feedback on my performance; maybe some things I needed to work on to improve my skills. But nothing was said and a couple more jobs came through which were thankfully straightforward.

Christmas came and went and then New Year's Day 2001 got off to a very fine start. A full English breakfast followed a laid back, lazy morning. As a family, we weren't big drinkers so New Year's Eve was a relatively sedate affair involving Big Ben on the television and singing Auld Lang Syne, but I treasured the fact that we were able to celebrate together. Many times over the previous few years my nursing shifts had kept me at the hospital, and on more than one occasion, I had actually been resuscitating someone as the bells chimed in the New Year. But now as I was working as an In-Flight nurse, repatriations were paused for a few days so I had the luxury of being at home.

As mentioned I was still living with my Mum and Dad at this point which benefited us all. I got a safe, secure base to return to in between trips without having to worry about the house standing empty whilst I was away; Mum and Dad got help with the bills and the security of knowing I was about if they needed anything. Mum's asthma had continued to plague her for many years, sometimes landing her in hospital, so Dad found it reassuring to have me dropping in and out on a regular basis. There was also the added bonus of being able to share in the pleasure of their dogs as it would have been impossible for me to have one of my own with being away so much. Although some people might think it not ideal to be still living with your parents as an adult, it worked well for us and was a win-win situation.

And to this day I cherish the luxury of not having to work a night shift on New Year's Eve anymore!

But although the repatriations were paused for a couple of days, Julie from the office was still on call so at 11am the phone rang. I smiled to myself as I answered: it had become a bit like Pavlov's dogs with the ringing of the phone triggering a quickening pulse and a surge of excitement.

She was organizing the repatriation of a lady named Jenny from Antigua. Would I be happy to fly out on the 3rd of January to go and collect her? The prospect of a trip to the warm and sunny West Indies in the middle of a cold and wet British winter sounded very enticing.

Once again, I had to pinch myself to believe that this was really my job. Some days I just couldn't believe my luck and was so grateful that I had been given the opportunity to do this. The only real down side it had was that I was employed on a free-lance basis so only got paid for the days I was actually on a job. A quiet spell would mean no income. I managed to get around this and make the job viable by signing up with a nursing agency so that I could do some shifts at my local hospitals if needed. This also had the advantage of allowing me to maintain my hospital skills. In practise, though, for a good two year period I found myself with more than enough trips to keep me busy. Working on repatriations also enabled me to save some money as all my expenses were paid whilst travelling, and being home so little of the time meant I didn't get much opportunity to socialise, shop or spend much. I had decided to just seize the opportunity and make the most of it without worrying about the financial side of it too much. As long as I had enough income to pay my bills then the benefit of the experiences I was having far outweighed monetary considerations.

So of course I said yes I would go to collect Jenny and two days later was sitting on a Virgin Atlantic flight from Heathrow to Antigua. It sounded like, and I hoped, that this would be another enjoyable and straight forward job.

Cheerful, melodic steel drums played us into the arrivals hall and as I made my way outside to the taxi rank, the delicious smell of tropical flowers swirled around in the breeze. It was warm and sunny and bright – such a contrast to the drizzled over London I had just left.

The next taxi in line was a battered old brown four-door saloon car. As soon as I approached, the driver's door popped open and a small, slim older gentleman wearing a brown leather flat cap and a gaudy floral shirt appeared in front of me. A huge smile spread across his face revealing perfect white teeth that seemed almost too big for his face. He held out his hand.

"I am Uncle Duncan," he said, in a lilting, sing-song voice that totally matched my image of a Caribbean accent. "Let me take your bag."

His warm and friendly manner endeared him to me straight away but I wondered if his car would even make it to the end of the street let alone to my hotel. Surprisingly, given its outward appearance, the inside was spotlessly clean, although it was dated and obviously very well used. I settled back in the tan-coloured leather seat and looked for the seat belt – there wasn't one, but there was a small floral cushion for my arm which was a thoughtful touch.

Uncle Duncan stowed my rucksack in the boot and then strolled around to the driver's seat. A minute or two passed as he got himself comfortable. Then the radio was twiddled into life, his flat cap adjusted and his car keys fished out of his pocket. It took me a minute to work out why the radio worked without the key in the ignition: it was a small portable transistor stuck onto the dashboard with some Blue Tac. It looked older than the car but it too had obviously been looked after as 'You Ain't Nothing But a Hound Dog' drifted clearly through to the back seat. After a few tries the car spluttered into life with an alarming rattling sound from under the bonnet that drowned out Elvis's hound dog. Uncle Duncan revved the engine a couple of times, adjusted his mirror and then off we trundled.

This was the start of things to come. I soon realised that a slow, relaxed pace was very much the way of life on the island. Everyone seemed to have the attitude that things would happen when they happened, and if they didn't happen at all, well, that was just fine as well. As the song says, it was very much, 'Don't Worry, Be Happy'. It took some time adjusting to this as we in the UK are all so used to being busy, busy, busy. At first, frustration got the better of me and I did a bit of huffing and puffing, but in the end I grew to quite like it. Ordering food turned out to be especially interesting – I learned quickly to order my meal at least an hour before I actually wanted to eat and to always have a book with me to while away the time spent waiting. That said, the food was delicious – a real triumph of culinary skill that expertly blended spices and colours together to make meals that wear as attractive as they were tasty.

Some minutes later the car rattled up to the front of a small, plain looking hotel set back from the road with just a blue hand painted sign announcing its name.

I waved goodbye to Uncle Duncan, who had obligingly offered to be my driver for the whole of the trip, and then made my way into the tiny lobby. The hotel was by no means grand but the view through the big picture window in reception took my breath away. What the building lacked in grandeur it more than made up for in location for it backed onto the most beautiful, classic, white-sand beach, so pristine in its whiteness it looked like something straight out of a tourism advert. I made a note to compliment Julie on her choice of hotels. Checking in involved a lengthy chat with the smiling lady on reception named Gladys and then she handed me a message to ring the office which I decided to do once I'd dropped my bag off and freshened up. Gladys pointed me out back towards my room.

Opening the door, I was delighted to see it faced the glorious beach with white wooden shutters at the window and a traditional ceiling fan that looked like a prop from a 1940s film. I almost expected Humphrey Bogart to stroll out of the bathroom with a cigarette in his mouth and a whiskey in his hand. Its charm was completed by the fact the windows had no glass in them so even with the shutters closed I could hear the sea.

Half an hour later, I made my way back to reception to call Julie. It makes me smile to think that now I would just whip out my mobile. Then, I had to wait whilst Gladys organised the call, and then Julie and I soon became aware that Enid, the operator at the telephone exchange, was on the call with us and kept joining in for a chat. It turned out that there had been a problem with the airline and our planned return flights had been cancelled. It would now be the 6th January before we could fly out. That meant I had two whole days free in Antigua before leaving for home. What a hardship – not! This was turning into a very nice trip and I couldn't help but feel a glow of anticipation spreading through me. Maybe I was about to experience a little bit of glamour after all and visions of that dreamy, white sand beach floated happily around my head.

Evening was fast approaching by this time so I quickly asked Enid to put in a call for me to my patient, Jenny. We arranged to meet up the following morning so that I could fill her in on our travel plans. She had had a severe asthma attack but was now doing very well and had been discharged from hospital. Because she had only recently been discharged, she needed a nurse with her on the flight to satisfy the airline's requirements and be certified as fit to fly. Her travel insurance paid for this and the repatriation company provided the staff: me. Strangely though she gave her address as a berth in English Harbour – she must be on a boat I surmised but gave it no more thought.

Dinner was a thoroughly entertaining affair that evening as the Trade Winds turned up. I had read about the Trade Winds and listened to romantic ballads about them over the years so naively imagined a gentle breeze blowing through my hair as I strolled on that idyllic white sand beach. The reality was that they were almost hurricane force. My whole evening was spent in the hotel's small outdoor courtyard restaurant – the indoor restaurant was closed for refurbishment - trying to stop my table blowing away and picking sand out of my eyes. Luckily, it was warm and the staff friendly and happy. Whiling away the three hours it took for my food to arrive, I saw the towering palm trees lining the beach still had red and green Christmas tinsel wrapped around their trunks. It was my first experience of being somewhere tropical over the festive season and the juxtaposition of sun, sea and sand with tinsel was surreal – definitely a strange sight.

The Trade Winds also proved to be problematic when I went to bed. They mercilessly smashed the window shutters around in their frames creating such an almighty racket that sleep was impossible. And the slats in the shutters allowed the mischievous winds to gain entry to my room and taunt me with their childish antics. They knocked over a potted plant, shook my bathroom door and did their best to rip my sheet off me. It was like having a poltergeist in the room. Eventually I admitted defeat and headed back to reception to see if I could change rooms. Thankfully the hotel was half empty so they gave me an inland room with a proper glass window. I was disappointed to lose that wonderful view of the beach and the sea but I needed some sleep.

But still it wasn't to be.

Once in my new quarters, a fresh torment made itself known: mosquitoes. Gleefully, they started dive-bombing me. There was no net so I spent the whole night cocooned from head to toe in the bed sheet – absolutely melting in the heat - but at least I was relatively safe from the little blighters. Sleep, sadly, still eluded me though as their incessant droning continued for most of the night. Who knew that Antigua even had mosquitoes? I did now.

The next morning the Trade Winds had moved off to torment someone else leaving a glorious sunny day with a sky so blue it looked like it had been polished. After an early breakfast, I found Uncle Duncan sat waiting for me at the front of the hotel.

"Where to, Miss Wendy?" he asked, beaming a huge smile that lit up every inch of his craggy face and seemed to be his default expression.

"English Harbour," I replied, returning his smile with one of my own.

"Aahh," he said, pulling open the back door of the car for me. "You will like it there."

He was right. I did like it. Very much.

The harbour, surrounded by lush green trees, sparkled into view as we approached. Gleaming, expensive yachts sat by the quayside whilst a myriad of small sailing boats dotted the deep blue water like tantalising sweets on the top of a cake. It looked like every detail had been brushed on with a delicate hand; care taken to create the red and yellow sails standing vibrantly against the cornflower blue sky, with just the occasional hint of cloud whisping by. Looking down on it brought a giddy sense of excitement; it was utterly gorgeous.

Then as we pulled up at the location Jenny had given me I couldn't quite believe what I was seeing. Moored at berth 11 was a vintage yacht complete with masts, towering sails, and a gleaming wooden hull that grabbed the sun and threw it back like dazzling jewels. Dwarfing everything around it, it appeared to pre-date all the other yachts by a good many years. I had seen some beautiful old ships before but never a yacht like this and never so close up. It truly was a sight that grabbed hold of the senses and left you breathless.

Uncle Duncan opened the car door for me and for the next couple of minutes we both stood transfixed as we admired her. Then I heard a voice call my name and looked up to see a smiling young woman dressed in white shorts and t-shirt with a deep tan almost the same colour as the teak deck.

"Jenny?" I called back.

"Yes, that's me. Come aboard."

It turned out that Jenny was crewing on the ship for the winter season as it sailed its way around the islands of the West Indies and the Caribbean. They were picking up and dropping off paying guests on their way; some spending a week on board whilst others just joined for a weekend of sailing.

Unfortunately though, Jenny had had a severe asthma attack. None of her usual medications or inhalers had given her any relief and she had then gone into status asthmaticus – a severe, prolonged asthma attack that had necessitated her urgent admission to hospital. This condition can be life threatening as the continuous fighting for breath puts a tremendous strain on the heart and can bring on a cardiac arrest. She had been very poorly but luckily had responded quickly to the emergency treatment she had been given. After a couple of days in hospital she had been allowed to return to the ship whilst it was in dock. However, it had been decided to not risk allowing her to continue with the next leg of the voyage hence the reason for me being there to take her home. She was understandably gutted to be cutting short her trip but had accepted it was the wisest decision.

I walked slowly up the gang way towards her, taking in the shining chrome, the polished deck and the sheer size of the masts and sails which soared above me like skyscrapers. This was definitely not the kind of ship I had expected her to be on.

"Come on," she said brightly, "I'll take you to meet the Captain."

Up close, a heaviness in her eyes gave away the fact that she had been poorly, but otherwise she looked well and definitely younger than her supposed forty two years.

I followed her through a door way and she led me down a maze of narrow corridors toward the ship's mess. At a small table, drinking coffee and reading a newspaper, sat a stocky grey haired man with a big bushy beard. It was all I could do not to start humming the tune from the fish-finger advert as a closer match to Captain Birdseye would have been hard to find. Smiling, he introduced himself as Geoff and he even seemed to have a mischievous twinkle in his eye just like the man on the television. I rather suspected that he was well aware of the similarity and playing up to the role for a bit of fun. In a deep, rumbling voice that perfectly matched his salty-sea-dog appearance he then invited us to join him for cake and coffee. We had no sooner slid onto the bench seat opposite, than the ship's cook delivered a big silver platter full of carrot cake and a fresh pot of steaming coffee. Carrot cake and coffee in the mess of a beautiful vintage yacht – this was definitely a first, and although not featuring a plane, I knew Dad was going to enjoy hearing about this particular trip.

We chatted about pleasantries for a few minutes and then I outlined our travel plans home explaining that our original flight had been cancelled and we now couldn't actually leave until the 6th – 2 days away.

The Captain looked slowly across at me and raised his eyebrows.

"Well, it just so happens," he said, "that we are not picking up our next lot of guests until the 6th so we have a free day tomorrow as well. Would you like to join us for a day of sailing around the Island?"

Once again, I couldn't believe my luck and didn't really need to answer as my stupid grin told him that it was a yes. Half an hour later I was heading back down the gang way with arrangements made to return at 9am the next day for the thrilling adventure that would be a day spent sailing around Antigua. What a treat that would be. Maybe I would concede that this classed as just a little bit glamorous!

On the quay side below I could see Uncle Duncan stretched out in the driver's seat of his battered jalopy waiting for me. I glanced at my watch and as it was still early I decided to ask him to take me on a tour of the island for the afternoon. He happily agreed but insisted I go to his house for lunch first to meet his mum and family. It seemed I was going to be well fed on this trip!

Setting off towards his home, I was taken aback by the poverty as we left the tourist part of the island. Most of the houses looked like little more than one room shacks and, just like Kathmandu, the streets were full of little children washing themselves under hosepipes and using the gutter as a toilet. The contrast was very sobering after the stunning beauty of English Harbour with its expensive yachts and swish cruise ship terminal lined with designer shops. I did briefly wonder if heading into this part of town in a taxi was a good idea. I had had the scare of my life down that back alley in Kathmandu – was I about to make yet another stupid mistake? But Uncle Duncan was chattering on, telling me about his sister who lived in the USA, and I liked him very much. The fact it was the middle of the day and bright and sunny also gave me confidence. I decided to put the thought out of my head and go with the flow. If any problems arose I would deal with them as and when needed.

Once or twice, Uncle Duncan stopped smack bang in the middle of the road and climbed out of the car to go and get one friend or another to say hello to me. They were all older men wearing the same flat cap as him, but all were unfailingly polite and happy to see me. By the time we reached his house I felt like some visiting member of the Royal family.

But then it got even more surreal.

Standing in the tiny front garden of the whitewashed bunga-low was Uncle Duncan's family, all waiting patiently to welcome me. There was his mum, two sisters, three brothers, an assort-ment of nieces and nephews, and a donkey named Elvis! I didn't know where to look first as they all crowded around me want-ing to give me hugs and talk to me. The women and children were all festooned in vivid yellows, oranges and pinks and it was like being swallowed by a rainbow. The men once again were all wearing the same brown flat caps as Uncle Duncan as if it were some kind of uniform, but their shirts shouted out in the same clash of colours as the women's dresses. Even Elvis the donkey wore a yellow bandana as he too clammered for my attention, pushing up behind me and nuzzling my hand. It was a complete and total sensory overload but I have never felt so welcome any-where in my entire life – it was like they had known me forever, but I was slightly puzzled as to how they knew we were coming.

Eventually, I had said hello to them all and was led around the house to a lawned area of grass that was bigger than the front garden but not by much. After my experience in Kathmandu I was unsure about eating their food in case they too had gone without in order to feed me. But there was a mountain of curries, breads, fruits and sweets so it seemed this wasn't the case. In comparison to most of the other families I'd seen on the journey here, it looked as if Uncle Duncan and his family were quite well off.

Two hours later I was stuffed full of food and almost one of the family. They were such friendly, warm people; it was a pleasure to spend time with them. And Elvis the donkey was happily letting me tickle his ears. He apparently lived in their little back garden but generally didn't get on with strangers so I was highly honoured that he appeared to like me as much as everyone else did.

With some difficulty, I managed to persuade Uncle Duncan it was time to leave. I think he was rather hoping we would just stay there all day, but as much as I had enjoyed meeting his family, I didn't want to miss my chance to see a little of the island.

After many more hugs and kisses and clutching a bag of sweet treats pushed into my hand by his Mum, we finally headed off down the street, their waves and smiles sending me off on a cloud of happiness. I never did find out how they knew we were coming, and my curiosity was piqued by Uncle Duncan's Mum. How old was she? He looked to be at least in his sixties so she must have been well into her eighties, but you would never have known it as she was energetic and vibrant, a real powerhouse of a woman who was clearly the centre of her large and loving family. Uncle Duncan was clearly delighted we had all had such a good time and he chatted happily away, throwing himself into the role of tour guide with much gusto.

And what a tour it turned out to be. Taking me from one tropical beach to the next, he told me about the history of the island as we went, regaling me with tales of colourful characters and their daring-do adventures. He was a great story teller and it was obvious that he really loved his home and was proud of all the riches it had to offer. After a while, we stopped for an hour at Dickenson Bay, an idyllic sweep of sand and sparkling water, so I could sunbathe and relax for a bit whilst he waited patiently for me by the roadside.

By the time I returned to the car, I had had three business offers ranging from setting up a diving school with a couple of grinning Rastafarians to running a small jewellery stall with a young boy named George who looked about 12. I had treated myself to a small pearl necklace from George's stall – which was an upside down beer crate - and although I doubted they were real pearls (he assured me they were!) it was very pretty and made a lovely little souvenir. I also might have had a cheeky little Pina Colada from the beachside bar!

After a wonder around the shops in the cruise terminal, Uncle Duncan dropped me back at the hotel, exhausted but very happy. I had even managed to pick up some mosquito repellent so my night was a little more comfortable.

As I look back on these trips now it still amazes me how much I managed to pack in to the limited time I had before collecting my patients. I nearly always saw some of the place and it was a great way of getting a feel for whether I liked somewhere and would like to return on holiday. Although on one trip my turn-around time was three hours so I saw nothing other than the hospital and the airport. But this was the exception rather than the rule and I generally got at least one day to explore.

Setting sail on the yacht the next morning was like sailing into a painting: the calm sea and cloudless sky joined forces to produce such a perfect vista that it didn't look like it could possibly be real. I settled on a perch at the front of the ship and as we slid out of the harbour and into deeper water the wind whipped my hair away from my face and coloured my cheeks with a pink glow. We dipped up and down into the water, the motion steady and soothing, the gentle slapping of the water on the hull the only sound I could hear. I closed my eyes and breathed deeply, the air salty and tangy and nourishing. At that moment I felt on top of the world. I was exactly where I wanted to be, doing exactly what I wanted to do. Did life get any better than this?

A couple of hours drifted past. At one point a pod of dolphins joined us, riding our bow wave with such joy it was infectious. There must have been about twenty of them, all dipping and diving in unison, the water frothing with their sleek bodies and leaping energy. Jenny joined me to watch them and we both found ourselves smiling and laughing – it was impossible not to feel a sense of connection with these beautiful creatures. Having seen this spectacle many times on wildlife programmes, it surprised me though how different it was seeing it for real in the wild. And how much more intense it was. The emotions that suddenly arose out of nowhere caught me totally off guard, rolling through me with such intensity they brought me close to tears. I couldn't even tell you specifically why. It was just so moving, so visceral, the connection so intimate. I tried to commit every second to memory so that I could summon up their joy again and again in the future. To this day it remains one of my most favourite moments of all time.

The dolphins eventually headed off and we sailed on. Occasionally, another yacht would bob into view and we attracted lots of attention and happy waves from their crews. Sea birds swooped and swirled around us and it really did seem as if nature was doing her finest display for us. Rounding a headland, a white sandy cove appeared over on our left side and it turned out that this was to be our lunch spot. The captain told us we couldn't sail the big ship into the cove so at this point we had to shimmy down a ladder into the yacht's rigid inflatable boat that would take us to shore. Upon hearing this a little bit of trepidation started circling around me. I'm not, and never have been, very athletic. But in the spirit of the day I bottled my fear and went for it. Taking it slowly I edged my way down the ladder and then fell rather than jumped down into the boat. It wasn't as bad as I thought it would be but I was seriously worried about getting back up again when it was time to leave. Jeans are also not the most flexible of garments for clambering around in but they were all I had with me having not been expecting to be spending time on boats when I left home.

But the ride in the inflatable to the beach was exhilarating. Racing along, it bounced us along the waves spraying water everywhere. Hanging on for dear life, I was soaked through but happily joined in with Jenny yelling for us to go faster.

The cove was sheltered and sunny and the sand as fine and white as sugar crystals. And it was completely deserted, our own little piece of paradise. The ship's cook had accompanied us and he had brought along a portable barbeque. Before long it was sizzling with all sorts of goodies and once again I feasted on delicious Caribbean food followed by another huge slice of the carrot cake we had had the day before. Sunbathing afterwards the only thing I was slightly concerned about was whether any of the scattered rocks on the beach would have anything alive and poisonous beneath them. Jenny assured me it was fine and we spent a lovely hour stretched out on the sand, chatting and sipping cold juices from the cook's cool bag.

As we talked, Jenny told me she was a solicitor in her everyday life. To cope with the long hours and stresses of the family law that she practised, she liked to run and do yoga. She also liked to sail. This was the third time she had taken time off from her law practice to spend a season crewing on a yacht and she hoped to do many more. Listening to her talk about the mental clarity it brought along with huge physical benefits made me start to think about whether such a venture might be something I my-self would like to do. I vowed to look into it further once back home.

All too soon our idyllic picnic was over and we were bouncing back towards the ship. Getting back up the ladder was just as embarrassing as I feared it would be. I didn't have the strength in my arms to haul myself up from the RIB so ended up with the cook and his mate shoving my backside to get me up. Not at all dignified and definitely not my finest hour, but I eventually made it back onto the ship. I did get a bit of teasing from the lads but it was all good natured and I only went a little bit red!

I thanked 'Captain Birdseye' profusely before disembarking. He had gifted me a truly fantastic experience – one I will never forget. As ever, Uncle Duncan was stretched out in his car, waiting patiently on the quayside to take me back to my hotel. That night, I slept better than I had done for a long time, the dolphins whisking me away into their watery playground and my ears thrilling to the sound of their clicks and whistles. I even slept through the ever present drone of the mosquitoes.

Bright and early the next morning we picked Jenny up from the quayside and headed to the airport. Steel drums once again greeted us at the airport. Uncle Duncan gave me a massive hug and I gave him a generous tip. His help had been invaluable and one of the reasons I enjoyed Antigua so much; he had definitely earned his money. As we were turning away from the car to head into the terminal, he suddenly thrust a small envelope into my hand.

"For you, Miss Wendy," he said. "Open it later."

I smiled. "Thank you, I will," I replied, popping it carefully into the front of my rucksack.

There was one more treat in store for us. British Airways were flying us home and they surprised us with an upgrade to Business Class. What a lovely end to a lovely trip.

Settled into our comfortable seats, we were sipping pre-flight chilled glasses of juice when I remembered Uncle Duncan's envelope. Pulling it out of my rucksack I saw my name carefully written in a long, looping script on the front. It contained one piece of carefully folded paper. Opening it my eyes nearly fell out of my head. Uncle Duncan started off by saying that he thought I was a beautiful young lady. He then went on to say he thought we could have a 'very lovely' life together and that he would be honoured if I would return to Antigua and marry him! He would take care of me and make sure I didn't want for anything. His mother had given her blessing and she was happy for me to live at their house with him and the rest of the family.

Well, that was something I hadn't expected!

My friends were always kidding me about spending my days flirting with handsome pilots and dashing doctors. That was the Mills and Boon fantasy. But it seemed, as with most things, that the reality of it was a little different. The reality was an old man in a flat cap with a donkey named Elvis!

CHAPTER 8

Swifts and Swallows 1981

The swifts and swallows swooped and soared above my head like miniature World War Two Spitfires in a dog fight. There must have been thirty or forty of them, all racing across a sky that was such a deep blue it looked like it had been taken straight from a photograph. Whistling and calling, the boomerang-shaped swifts raced towards one another at breakneck speed, inherently knowing the precise moment to veer off and head back up towards the vast blueness. Again and again they circled round, their calls getting louder and louder and louder. I could see why this phenomenon is known as a 'screaming party'. The sight captivated me, my eyes zooming across the sky with them. I didn't want to miss a moment of their energy and joy. No winners, no losers, just life at full throttle. From being a little girl, their spring return was always an eagerly awaited spectacle, despite the fact that it fell near Andrea's anniversary. That day in May when they swooped in after their epic migration from Africa always brought happiness with it, a lifting of spirits that signalled the start of warmer weather and the blossoming colours of spring.

Today, it was a hot June day in 1981. The swifts and swallows had been with us about two weeks and I never tired of joining their party whenever one kicked off – often every day at the peak of the season. Beneath their whooshing wings, pink and yellow roses, their scent coaxed out by the warmth of the sun, gathered around the wooden bench I was sitting on. The garden of the home we had moved to when I was 13 was small, little more than a few square metres, but Mum had filled it with tubs of begonias and geraniums, dahlias and lilies, whilst clematis climbed the shed and smothered its roof with a confection of lilac flowers. In the corner, a small rabbit hutch that Dad had made was home to Caroline and Andrew's two black and white rabbits: Smokey and Sooty.

Dad came out to join me and I scooted over to make room for him on the bench beside me. I was eighteen-years-old and had just finished doing my A levels. The previous week had gifted me an interview to start nurse training at Bolton School of Nursing. I was waiting to hear if I'd been accepted.

Dad had in his hand a long white envelope. He held it out to me and a little ripple of nervous energy mixed in with a dollop of fear skittered up my spine as I saw the 'Bolton General Hospital' postmark. I didn't have a 'plan b'. My heart was set on being a nurse – if I didn't get in I didn't know what I would do instead.

I reached out and took the envelope. It was smooth, plain, nondescript – hard to imagine that something so unremarkable could hold something so important. But it did, it held my future. In just a few short seconds I would know.

Overhead, the swifts screamed past, their wings beating faster and faster, getting ever more frenzied as if they knew what an important moment this was and couldn't contain themselves.

Dad smiled his lop-sided smile. Always a handsome man, tall with hair so dark it was almost black, his smile seemed to make him glow with an inner warmth that always made people like him. In fact, I don't think I have ever met anyone who didn't sing his praises; old ladies in particular seemed to have lots of problems with their washing machines that needed his help to fix. Of course, he always happily obliged and Mum would roll her eyes as he disappeared yet again into some house or other to lend a hand. Over the years a little bit of his magic rubbed off on me and I was automatically liked and accepted as 'John's daughter' everywhere I went. His steady, solid presence made me feel safe. And now, his smile twinkled his blue eyes and reassured me.

Could my dream of being a nurse really be about to come true?

"Go on," he said, "open it."

Carefully, I turned the envelope over and eased open the flap. It contained a single piece of headed notepaper folded over three times. Pulling it out, I took a deep breath and opened it. The words, 'We are delighted to offer you . . .' jumped out at me. I looked up at Dad. He was grinning.

"Told you!" he said. "I knew you'd get in."

And in that moment, not only was I delighted that I was going to be a nurse, but I was also overwhelmed with gratitude that I had people who believed in me more than I believed in myself. I had people who loved me, I had succeeded in my A levels, and now I had my coveted place at Bolton School of Nursing. My emotions got the better of me and tears bubbled up, leaking down my face and stealing my voice. But by then Dad had his arm around me and was squeezing me in a tight bear hug. I hugged him back, my tears most definitely the happy kind.

That day with the swifts and swallows whooping their joy in the sky above me now seems to have taken on an extra dimension in my memory, to have become even more poignant. It feels as if it was a sign of things to come. That I would find great happiness and satisfaction in being a nurse. And that I would also get to soar into the great blue yonder myself.

CHAPTER 9

Cape Town

As a nurse you get used to keeping tight control of your emotions. It quickly becomes apparent that you are no use to your patients or their relatives if you can't maintain a calm, professional demeanour in the face of heartbreak and sadness. Patients need you to look after them and they need you to be there for and support their loved ones. Often, they are having the worst day of their lives; you can't always change that, you can't work miracles. But what you can do is be a calm, reassuring presence. You can talk to them and soothe them. You can ensure they are kept fully informed about what's happening. And you can empathize with them and let them know you understand and care about them.

But keeping a calm appearance doesn't mean you don't sometimes feel intense emotions, only that you have become adept at controlling them in order to do your job well. When the shift is over, sometimes those emotions can hit you like a baseball bat. On many occasions over the years I have been driving home when the tears have come. It's not a bad thing or a sign of weakness. It releases those very real feelings and it means you are a human being that cares. Personally, I think if that stops happening and you become hardened to the suffering of your patients, then maybe it is time to look for a different job.

And there are undeniably some patients who will affect you in a more profound way than others. Their story will burn its way into your memory creating a permanent scar. You will be forever changed by them. Sometimes this will be in a good way for they have taught you valuable lessons and helped you mature and grow in both your career and your personal sense of self. But other times it will be in a negative way that shocks you and forces you to confront the cruelty that exists in the world, the tragedies that befall people and how unfair life can be.

One such case I will never forget is that of three-year-old Alfie.

He was beaten to death by his father because he was splashing too much water about when he was having a bath. I deliberately don't use the term 'Daddy' as in my view no one who does that to a child can ever be called their 'Daddy'.

The man yanked Alfie by his ankles out of the bath and swung him head first into the bathroom wall. He then dropped him onto the floor and stamped on him.

Fourteen stone against a three-year-old. One of the lasting images I have of that little boy is the perfect size ten boot print that was emblazoned across his back.

Alfie's Mum was downstairs hoovering at the time so she didn't hear the commotion upstairs. The first she knew something had happened was when she heard the front door slam as Alfie's father stormed out of the house. Hearing only silence from upstairs and starting to panic she ran up to investigate and found Alfie.

He was blue-lighted to the Paediatric Intensive Care Unit I was working on at the time and placed on a ventilator. Three hours later he died.

I gently washed his broken body and dressed him in his favourite Thomas the Tank Engine t-shirt. I combed his hair, carefully arranging it to hide the blood. Then I held his Mum, Sarah, in my arms as she screamed. I filled in paperwork and liaised with the police officers that were guarding the unit in case his father turned up. They were looking for him but were unable to find him.

My professional self guided me through one of the most difficult shifts of my career. Then I went home and sobbed. I will never forget little Alfie and the man who did that to him. I believe he was sent to prison for thirteen years.

Another case that was very different but no less memorable was that of Ralph. He was a strong, fit twenty-eight-year old that had gone to Cape Town with his mates for a stag do. Unfortunately for Ralph he had a heart problem that he knew nothing about. In the back of a taxi on his way to the party, he suffered a cardiac arrest. His heart stopped dead and he keeled over on to the floor. Luckily, he was with two of his friends and they immediately started CPR and alerted the taxi driver. He sped them towards the nearest hospital. Unluckily, the traffic that evening was very heavy and the hospital was some distance away. It took them over fifteen minutes to get there. As mentioned previously, even if you do CPR perfectly as a trained medical professional, much less oxygen gets to the brain than normally would. Ralph was rushed into the Emergency Room and given top class medical care. But he had been down over twenty minutes by this point and his brain was severely starved of oxygen. His friends had undoubtedly saved his life – if they hadn't been there, he would have died in the back of the taxi – but he was left severely brain damaged.

After several weeks in Intensive Care in Cape Town, the decision was made to bring him home to the UK to continue his recovery. I met Tom at Heathrow to fly out and go get him.

As with Mavis, we were taking all the equipment we would need with us so we had a cardiac monitor, portable ventilator, portable suction, bag of drugs and a scoop stretcher. This type of stretcher is two long metal halves that slot together; you slide one half under each side of the patient and then fasten it together. It makes it possible to get the patient on and off the stretcher more easily and is the same one mountain rescue teams use. It's bulky to transport but less so than other forms of stretchers. Luckily, there were two of us to see to everything on this trip and we checked it all into the hold before we boarded.

What happens when you are bringing a patient back on a stretcher on a commercial flight is that the airline engineers collapse down several rows of seats on one side at the back of the aircraft. This provides a flat platform that the stretcher can then be bolted to keep it secure for the duration of the flight. It can sometimes be a little disconcerting for the patient as the stretcher is quite high up and near to the curved top of the plane – they can also feel a little claustrophobic. The accompanying staff are given a row of seats in the centre aisle across from the patient. Patient and staff are pre-boarded before the rest of the passengers to give time to get the stretcher anchored in place and the patient settled before take-off. Often times there could be problems for the engineers securing the stretcher, and we have on occasion unfortunately delayed departure, but luckily this didn't happen with Ralph. But first we had to go and collect him from the hospital.

After a meal and overnight rest in a hotel, Tom and I loaded our not inconsiderable equipment into a taxi and headed to the hospital. The scoop stretcher was our biggest item to transport but taking our own made things much easier in the long run as once Ralph was secure on it he wouldn't need to come off it again until we reached the UK hospital he was being admitted to.

Once on the unit, two staff handed over to us and then I helped them change Ralph and get him ready for the journey. He was, to put it simply, in a very bad way. Unable to breath properly for himself he had a tracheostomy in his throat connected to 100% oxygen via a t-tube and a piece of flexible tubing. A feeding tube provided fluids and nutrition as he was unable to eat and drink, and he was doubly incontinent so needed a urine catheter and nappy-style pads. He was also very confused and agitated and appeared to have no idea what was happening to him or what was going on. Apart from the fact that it was extremely sad to see such a young man in such a state, it also meant the journey home was going to be a challenging one. Drugs would be given as and when necessary in an attempt to keep him calm, but with a brain insult this is fraught with difficulty and needs great care. Ralph pulling out his tracheostomy, feeding tube or catheter was a serious concern and we would need to be hypervigilant to stop him doing this. Not only could he hurt himself, but it would also be very difficult to deal with at 38000 feet in the confines of an aircraft.

I chatted away quietly to him as we worked in an attempt to settle him and get him used to my voice. Although his deep brown eyes were pools of fear, and he looked at me in complete incomprehension, he did seem to rest a little easier and didn't fight us as we changed him. Once loaded into the ambulance for the short run to the airport, Tom and I discussed what we would need to do to keep Ralph as comfortable and safe as possible. Ralph also had pneumonia so top of the list would be sucking out the secretions from his tracheostomy to keep his chest as clear as possible thereby ensuring a steady supply of oxygen actually got down into his lungs. Intravenous antibiotics would need to be given along with regular pain relief.

Unfortunately, as we were loading him onto the plane and securing the stretcher in place, he began to get more and more agitated. This was not altogether unexpected as the stimulation of what was going on would be difficult for his fragile brain to process. The noise and the people and the movement were just overwhelming for him.

There was a small privacy curtain to pull around him during the flight but sadly it did little to actually keep things private. Lots of eyes stared at us as the other passengers boarded and his distress was plain for everyone to see.

Tom gave him a sedative via his intravenous line and I held his hand and stroked his arm in an attempt to sooth him. He calmed down a little but I ended up spending much of the flight holding his hands, both to comfort him and to stop him pulling his various tubes out. These tubes into the throat and bladder often cause some degree of discomfort so confused patients can become preoccupied with yanking them out in order to remove the strange sensations.

Sucking out his tracheostomy and keeping his airway clear also proved to be a huge challenge. We were using a thin, flexible tube connected to our suction machine. When Ralph's respirations became bubbly we would feed the tube down into Ralph's lungs and draw out the secretions that were threatening to block his wind pipe. But our portable suction machine was struggling with the horrible, thick green pneumococcal mucus he was producing – they are a handy little machine but nowhere near as powerful as the full-sized ones found in hospitals. There was also the fact that the container that caught the secretions was small and filled up rapidly; emptying it and washing it out in the tiny toilet cubicle was tricky as it wouldn't fit under the tap. This sucking out process is also deeply unpleasant for the patient as it makes them cough and feel as if they are choking. In Ralph's agitated state it made things much more uncomfortable for him and caused his distress to shoot up.

The worst thing by far was seeing the tormented, haunted look in his eyes; fear flitted around behind them giving him the appearance of a hunted animal that knew a predator was closing in. Nothing we did seemed to come anywhere close to easing that for him. He had been a strong, fit young man who ran marathons, but now he was trapped in a body already showing signs of muscle wastage. His skin had yellowed over and taken on a pale and sallow tone. He looked so much older than his twenty eight years. When I looked at him, I could imagine my brother lying there – what a terrible tragedy. And I suppose it could be said that the predator he feared had already ambushed him.

It also transpired that Ralph had a wife and six-year-old little boy waiting for him at home. They were going to meet us at Heathrow and then travel by road with us, following our ambulance to the hospital. His wife had been out to Cape Town to visit him but his little boy, Jack, had not seen his Daddy since he had been taken poorly several weeks before. It was going to be a tremendous shock for that child to see his Daddy like this; the last time he had seen him he had been fit, well and smiling as he headed off at the airport. I had my doubts that doing this first meeting in the back of an ambulance at Heathrow was a good idea, but that was what his wife wanted so Tom had reluctantly agreed.

The flight droned on in a predictably long and tiring way. It is very draining caring for a confused and agitated patient so Tom and I took it in turns caring for Ralph so that the other could eat and take little breaks. A very kind flight attendant named Jill kept us supplied with coffee and nibbles and did her best to give us as much space as possible. Once again, I was glad to have Tom with me, not only because of his medical skill and ability to share Ralph's care, but also because of the steady, calm manner that seemed to be his trademark. Nothing seemed to faze him. Ralph constantly trying to pull out his tracheostomy and catheter started to wear me down but having Tom to chat to kept the atmosphere light and easy-going and enabled me to cope with it much more easily. When he could see me getting tired he stepped in with a comment or two that broke the tension and pressed my reset button. It was definitely a team effort that got us through the long hours of the flight and safely back to London.

Unfortunately, on landing at Heathrow, Tom got an urgent message.

"I have to go," he said. "Will you be okay doing the road journey on your own?"

I nodded. "Yes, no problem."

But I have to admit that my heart sank. The prospect of managing Ralph, all our equipment, and Ralph's family all on my own was more than a little daunting. Tiredness had already got a hold of me after the long flight and it becomes harder to muster up the level of patience needed to care for such a patient when you are exhausted. But, it had to be done. This was my job and what I had signed up for, so I organised myself and got on with it. My professional self once more rose to the challenge and guided me onwards, but lurking as ever at the back of my mind was that nagging inner voice. "Here we go," it taunted, "this is when you really mess it up."

The hydraulic lift off loaded us from the aircraft with no problems and two paramedics whisked us straight over to our ambulance that was waiting on the tarmac. They quickly and efficiently loaded the stretcher in to the back of the vehicle. The British weather was throwing rain and a cold wind at us which seemed to fit the sombre mood that accompanied us. Tom checked Ralph over and then, happy that he was safe to continue on the journey, he said his goodbyes and left us.

One of the paramedics, Kieran, climbed in the back of the ambulance with me and told me that Ralph's wife, Mandy, and his son were already there and waiting patiently for us to call them round. I did my best to make Ralph as presentable as possible. I wrapped an extra blanket around him to cover his feeding tube and catheter but there was little I could do about his tracheostomy and oxygen tubing and the deep rasping sounds that the pneumonia was producing in his chest as he breathed. I hoped the little boy wouldn't be too frightened when he saw his Daddy.

When we were ready, or as ready as we were ever going to be, Kieran went to get them and I held Ralph's hand as we waited. Almost as if he knew something momentous was about to happen, Ralph seemed to melt into the pillows and the tension that had been hovering over him throughout the whole of the journey appeared to soften and dissipate. His hand relaxed in mine and the rattling in his chest even came down a notch. I closed my eyes and took a few deep breaths myself. I didn't know how this meeting would go but I guessed it might be hard all round.

After a few minutes, there was a gentle tap and the ambulance door slowly opened to reveal a young dark-haired woman dressed in jeans and a navy blue padded coat. Standing just behind her, clutching her hand tightly and looking down at the floor, was Jack. I knew he was six-years-old but he looked younger. Mandy was putting on a brave face for her little boy and she murmured soothingly to him as she turned and scooped him up in her arms. She locked eyes with me, nodded, and then slowly carried Jack up the steps and into the ambulance. Kieran closed the door behind her and we were left with the dim light of the grey day through the window and the smell of wet clothes.

Ralph's confusion still smothered him; when Mandy said his name there was no reaction and he didn't appear to recognize her. She gently put Jack down at the side of the stretcher. At first he continued to stare fixedly at his trainers, but then, after a moment of hesitation, he slowly lifted his head and looked straight at his Daddy. Shock widened his eyes but he was so brave and didn't cry or turn away. After a few seconds, he tentatively reached out for Ralph's hand and said simply, "Hello, Daddy, it's me, Jack."

For a moment silence hung in the back of the ambulance as if it too was holding its breath. Waiting and watching. All that could be heard was the rattling of Ralph's chest and the rain drumming its fingers on the window. Then Ralph turned his head slowly towards his little boy. And we all saw it. The exact moment recognition flared in his eyes. And then he started to cry.

Incredibly, Ralph fought off the pneumonia and after twelve weeks in hospital was transferred to a specialist rehabilitation unit. Many months of hard work later, he was finally well enough to go home with Mandy and Jack. Their house was adapted to cope with his extra needs and he continued to progress slowly but steadily. Today, he walks with a stick and has some memory issues, but he is able to work part time from home.

And the best news?

He and Mandy had another baby boy so Jack got to be a big brother!

CHAPTER 10

Mallorca

A gentle tap sounded on my hotel door and then a soft Scottish voice drifted through: "Wendy, it's me, Maggie. Have you got another five Euros for a wee cup of tea?"

My eyes rolled heavenward as I tried, and failed, to stop myself groaning. It was 11pm and this was the third time in two hours that Maggie had been to my door for 'Euros for a wee cup of tea'. Earlier in the day I had learned that her 'wee cups of tea' were in fact ninety percent whiskey with a drop of Earl Grey to colour them brown. What type of whiskey didn't seem to concern her, just as long as it had a hefty alcohol content. And what time of day it was also didn't seem to bother her. I like to think of myself as being an easy-going person but by this point the thread that tethered me to my patience was stretched to its limit and almost ready to break. I did however find a grudging smile flitting across my face: it was safe to say that the set of circumstances that Maggie found herself in were making her very happy indeed.

A retired lady in her late sixties from Glasgow, on the surface Maggie looked like your average older lady with a penchant for sensible shoes and comfortable trousers topped with pink knitted jumpers and a short grey perm. She was quick to smile, quick to laugh and always had her black patent leather handbag draped over her arm reminiscent of the Queen.

Enjoying a late winter holiday in Mallorca with her friend Agnes, they had been sunbathing by the hotel pool when Agnes had suddenly collapsed. There was no warning: she had gone from relaxing on her sun lounger to unconscious within seconds. It was found that she was in a very fast heart rhythm – a condition where the heart is firing off rapid electrical impulses that are both chaotic and ineffective at producing an efficient heartbeat to deliver blood around the body. Her heart needed to be shocked back into a normal rhythm using a defibrillator. Agnes fortunately had a guardian angel looking out for her that day as the hotel staff were trained in first aid and had acted quickly. Paramedics had arrived and got her to the local hospital in record time. After cardio-verting her heart back to a normal rhythm with the defibrillator, they had then operated and fitted an internal pacemaker. This is a small device inserted under the skin on the chest that kicks in if the arrhythmia happens again, hopefully preventing further collapse. Progressing well following this procedure, she had been deemed fit to fly with a nurse – me – and her companion – Maggie. Oxygen had been booked for her on the plane in case she needed it in transit. This is always booked as extra to what the plane would normally carry and had been arranged by Julie when the flights were booked.

Collecting the ladies from the hospital went smoothly and we arrived at the airport check-in with time to spare. But then the first problem of the day made itself known: something had gone wrong during the booking process and there was no oxygen available on the flight for us. We were shown to a waiting area whilst they tried to sort it out. An hour crawled by and we were still waiting. Then they started boarding all the other passengers. Departure time was fast approaching and still we waited.

Eventually, a customer care agent from the airline came rushing over to us. The look on her face said that it was not good news. They couldn't get any extra oxygen on board the flight in time and therefore the only way we could fly was to go without it. That was not something we could risk. If Agnes became ill on the flight she would most definitely need oxygen; she was doing well but we couldn't be sure that the reduced oxygen levels in the cabin wouldn't affect her. The agent duly told us that the captain agreed that we couldn't risk it and had therefore decided we couldn't fly. Our seats would have to be rebooked onto a later flight.

Back at the ticket desk, more bad news awaited us. School half term week had just started so all the flights were fully booked for the next few days; the earliest flight they could get us on was in five days time. This was obviously less than ideal.

I sat the ladies down back in the waiting area and went off to call Julie at the office. Should I take Agnes and Maggie back to the hospital? It turned out they wouldn't accept Agnes back as she had been discharged and didn't need to be in hospital. It was decided that the best course of action was to take the flights for five days time and in the meantime check us all into the hotel that I had stayed in the night before. The heat had been building steadily as the day progressed so by this time we were all hot and fed up and Maggie was complaining that she was thirsty. Bottles of water didn't do it for her; she wanted a wee cup of tea.

A taxi whisked us back over to the hotel, its air conditioning providing a welcome break from the blazing heat. Luckily, they had rooms available which given that it was half term was very fortunate indeed. Checking the three of us in, we had one room for me and one room for Agnes and Maggie, just down the hall from each other. Julie authorised me to pay for whatever we needed and they would cover it. After dropping off our bags and a freshen up, we headed to the restaurant for dinner.

This was the point where I discovered that Maggie's 'wee cups of tea' were in fact mostly whiskey, and Maggie discovered that all their food and drink was being paid for. So she was 'stuck' in a nice four star hotel in Mallorca with unlimited food and drink all paid for. Agnes was subdued and tired as she had been poorly and it had been a long day, but Maggie, well, she thought all her birthdays had come at once.

And so dinner unexpectedly developed into a very lively affair. I thought a quiet meal and then an early night would be the order of the day. I was, after all, with two older ladies. But Maggie had other ideas.

We were sat at a table around the edge of a wooden dance

floor. Following our meal, a Spanish Flamenco dancer stepped into the middle of the floor and entertained us with her swishing scarlet red gown and flying feet. Then we entertained her when Maggie jumped up and decided to join in. Now Maggie most definitely did not have the grace or physique of a dancer. In fact she was a rather round lady who was little more than five feet tall and sort of bounded around more like a kangaroo than a dancer. Several times she almost crashed into the tables but miraculously she just about managed to stay on her feet. The poor dancer didn't know what to do and neither did I. Embarrassment dragged my gaze into my lap as I tried to deny that she was with Agnes and me. But, despite myself, I did end up snorting with laughter. After enjoying several 'wee cups of tea' Maggie was hilarious and certainly knew how to play to her audience. Within minutes she had the other diners all whooping and clapping and egging her on. She stamped her feet and twirled her hands, even joining in singing to the music at one point. I had to give her credit: her stamina for an older woman was enviable. Eventually she ran out of steam and the exhausting spectacle came to a thunderous close with Maggie getting loud cheers from everyone in the room. The poor dancer had by this time disappeared off the dance floor and left her to it.

Maggie took several bows before her adoring audience and then floated back to our table on a cloud of adrenaline and whiskey.

"Ready for bed?" I asked hopefully, surprised but relieved when she nodded and agreed to call it a night. But then she apparently changed her mind. After I left Maggie and Agnes at their room, unbeknown to me Maggie turned around and headed straight back down to the bar. She tried to charge her drinks to my room but the hotel staff wouldn't let her. And so began the little trips asking for money. I obliged a couple of times but it soon became apparent that Maggie intended taking full advantage of the situation. I rang the office to ask for advice and clarification as to how much of Maggie's bar bill they were willing to cover.

Julie had never encountered this before so went off to see what Tom wanted us to do. After a few minutes she rang me back, and unfortunately for me, said I should give them both whatever they wanted to keep them happy. My heart sank. It was going to be a long five days.

A cheap swimsuit from a local shop meant I was able to enjoy a bit of swimming and sunbathing, but this was punctuated by regular trips to the cash machine to get money for Maggie. I soon worked out that the only way to stop her knocking at my door until gone midnight was to give her a chunk of money each evening after we had eaten. This kept her very happy and gave me a bit of peace. Agnes, who was my actual patient, was no trouble what so ever. A quiet, softly spoken lady, she was happy to relax by the pool and drink actual tea – it was Maggie who was the handful!

This became our new routine until the end of the week when we were finally able to head back to the airport for our homeward flight. I had booked a wheelchair and was pushing Agnes to conserve her strength for the journey. Maggie, as an accompanying companion, was supposed to look after herself and was not legally my responsibility. If anything, family or friends that travelled with us were actually supposed to help me with the patient and their luggage. However, Maggie quickly made it known that she was not happy at Agnes being pushed in a wheelchair whilst she had to walk. A little rich considering her Flamenco antics a few days earlier! She started huffing and puffing and then the complaining began. Her legs were aching. She was tired. The heat was making her feel dizzy. To placate her I had to go and get her a wheelchair too. Unfortunately there were no customer care agents free to help me so I had to set up a relay system whereby I pushed Agnes, then parked her up with the bags and went back for Maggie. By the time we actually boarded our flight my legs were aching, I was tired and the heat was getting to me! I consoled myself with the fact that at least they had our oxygen and we had been allowed to board this time.

But this was just the first leg of the journey. The only flights we'd been able to get were Mallorca to Madrid, Madrid to Heathrow and then Heathrow to Glasgow, so a very long day of travelling loomed in front of us. Luckily, I managed to phone Julie at the office before we boarded and get her to organise a second wheelchair and a member of staff to help me at Madrid and Heathrow. This would at least help to make things a bit easier.

Much to my dismay, though, the excitement just kept coming. As is often the case with these trips, once problems start, they come thick and fast.

We sat on the aircraft waiting for pushback. And we waited. Then we waited some more. I said a silent prayer to anyone who would listen – please don't let us have to get off again because there's a problem with the aircraft. Another twenty minutes passed and then the Captain came on to make an announcement. Here we go, I thought, the plane is broken and we have to disembark. I breathed a sigh of relief when he said there had been an issue with the plane but it was now fixed and we would shortly be on our way. Fishing our tickets out to check them, my heart sank when I looked at our connection time in Madrid. The extended delay meant we had only minutes to get to our next flight. It was very unlikely that we would be able to make it with two wheelchairs. The possibility of getting stuck in Madrid loomed large and at that point I was very tempted to have one of Maggie's 'wee cups of tea'. (Several miniature bottles of whiskey from the hotel mini bar had mysteriously found their way into her handbag and she was already rustling up her first tea of the day. It then dawned on me why she always kept her bag held so closely to her side.)

The plane deposited us in Madrid ten minutes before our flight to Heathrow was due to depart. Never going to happen, I thought, as I resigned myself to having to stay in Spain for the night. But then the most fabulous thing happened that brightened my mood immensely. The Captain told everyone to stay seated as some passengers were being taken off the plane first . . . and those passengers were us! Two members of the ground crew came on board and whisked us off the plane. Two wheelchairs stood at the ready. It seemed our fully loaded connecting flight was sat on the tarmac waiting for us – they had delayed the flight!

The two lads propelled Agnes and Maggie across the transit lounge at breakneck speed with me running behind clutching our bags. It was hair raising watching them weaving in and out of the crowds but amazingly the ladies loved it whilst I was secretly relieved that I wouldn't have to spend another night on this job.

A sea of faces greeted us as we huffed and puffed our way onto the plane and then a wave of clapping and cheering washed down the aisles. I didn't know where to look I was so embarrassed. Perhaps predictably, Maggie was lapping up all the attention and seemed to be having a grand old time. I said another silent prayer of thanks that Agnes was well and seemed to be coping with all the stress without any problems – just as well really. I did allow myself a little snigger though when, after take-off, Maggie proclaimed loudly that she now definitely needed a wee cup of tea and the cabin crew apologized but said they had run out of tea and would coffee be ok. Her face was worthy of Instagram and I'm guessing that whiskey doesn't go so well with coffee!

Thankfully, the rest of that flight passed without incident and we all got to relax a little and recharge ready for our Heathrow transfer. I have to say Heathrow is not one of my favourite airports – it's nothing specific, just the general size and busyness of the place – so I'm always glad when I am through and seated on my flight out. But it does have nice lounges and there was one more treat waiting for Maggie.

Collecting our tickets at the British Airways desk, the agent smiled at us and presented us with Business Class tickets. Julie had booked them as they were the only flights available to Glasgow that day. With Business Class tickets comes the Business Class lounge and with the Business Class lounge comes . . . free alcohol. Maggie was delirious with happiness when we were escorted to the lounge and invited to help ourselves to whatever we wanted. Unbeknown to me, her handbag now contained more than a dozen empty miniature whiskey bottles. Quick as a flash she set off filling them from the dizzying array of spirits on offer. I may at the point have decided I urgently needed the toilet and disappeared for a little while!

Maggie provided a running commentary on the flight up to Glasgow telling anyone who would listen all about her day. With a few drinks firing her up, she was incredibly witty and entertaining and soon had the cabin crew giggling away. I'd started off rolling my eyes at her antics earlier in the week but by the time we were flying over the Clyde on our approach to Glasgow I had really started to enjoy her company. She was one sassy lady who knew how to have a good time! She and Agnes couldn't have been more different but I guess that's probably why they were such good friends: as they say, opposites attract. That said, I was still glad to hand them over to their families in Glasgow and make my way to my hotel for a little peace and quiet. It had been a hugely entertaining trip – if 'entertaining' is the right word – but it had been full on and exhaustion wound itself around my shoulders like coiled rope.

I arrived at the hotel at 7pm, had dinner, quietly and with no dancing, and then went to bed. It was so lovely to settle back on my pillows, safe in the knowledge that there wouldn't be any tap, tap, taps at my door. I never did find out exactly how much money Maggie's tea addiction cost the company but I'm sure it must have been quite a considerable amount. But I had fulfilled my brief: I had got them home safely and kept them both happy. Job done.

CHAPTER 11

Flying

My shiny new Registered General Nurse badge propelled me down the hospital corridor towards the job board. Ironed to within an inch of its life, my blue uniform dress fitted perfectly, and an expert military-style clean by my Dad had polished up my black shoes. We still wore hats then, and although it sounds a bit daft now, they were a source of great pride. I had been a qualified nurse for two whole days and many mixed emotions swirled around. But by far the most dominant one was elation - I had completed my training and had the whole of my career ahead of me. I felt lighter; the world different: brighter and more intense as if someone had turned up the contrast and made all the colours somehow pop out at me.

Getting a position after qualifying was very different back then to what it is now. When a group of student nurses qualified, a list of available jobs would be put up on the board. You would then choose which post you wanted and put your name down beside it on the list. If you were the only one who wanted that post, you were given it; if more than one person wanted the same one then you would be interviewed and the sister on that particular ward would choose who she wanted. The ones not chosen would then move on down their list of preferences until they got something that suited them. There were usually more jobs than nurses so everyone got something; not getting a job after qualifying was virtually unheard of. Sadly, that's not always the case now in our modern NHS, and you certainly cannot just pick a job and walk straight into it a few days later.

My eyes excitedly searched the list. There it was: Paediatrics. A job was available on the children's ward and so far no one else had put their name down. I carefully selected a black pen from the neat row of pens sitting in my top pocket, filled in my name, and then went home to begin the agonising wait. Two days later the news came that the job was mine. Much less red tape complicated things back then so I was just told to report to the ward the following Monday.

Mum and Dad were, of course, delighted for me. To celebrate, Dad cooked a massive roast dinner and Mum made my favourite Victoria sponge cake with great dollops of strawberry jam and oodles of fresh cream oozing out. Endless possibilities lit up my future and I felt happy and proud of myself for having achieved my goal. I had worked hard and I had done it. Youthful enthusiasm glowed on my face, shiny and new, just like my badge. And what a great thing that is. If only we could bottle that feeling to use in future years when times get tough and life events weigh us down.

A lot of people bemoan nursing as a hard and stressful job, which it undoubtedly is at times, but I will always be grateful for the opportunities that it has given me. I don't think there are many careers that can offer such variety, such satisfaction, such scope for growth and learning. It undeniably has its challenges but if you can cope with these the rewards are immense.

But, whilst Andrea's death was the catalyst that set me off towards working in Paediatrics when I qualified, it was also ultimately the thing that led to me giving it up.

B1 was a superb ward to work on and the kids were a joy to look after. But I couldn't cope when they died. The really sick children got to me. It was just too upsetting. When I was caring for them I could imagine Andrea in their place. At the time of her death my age protected me from most of the horrors of her illness, but now my job was filling in the blanks. Day by day I was putting together my own mental picture of what it must have been like. What she must have gone through. What my Mum must have gone through. I experienced every loss with such intensity. And it started to take its toll. Soon, the shininess dimmed and I began to dread going into work. My heart would drop like a stone when I was assigned one of the very poorly children to look after. Of course, I was getting more experienced so was able to maintain my professional front and not let my emotions show, but I had not yet reached the stage where I could process my feelings and deal with them in a healthy way. I was bottling it all up. Day by day, bit by bit. Gradually, realisation dawned that this speciality was not where my future lay. These children needed dedicated caring nurses to look after them but sadly, I couldn't be one of them.

The final straw came when I was caring for a two-year-old little boy named Jed who had had abdominal surgery. Unsettled and crying, his Dad had picked him up to try and soothe him. He had him over his shoulder and was patting his back gently when I walked into the sideward.

"He's settled now," Dad said, giving me a tired smile. "He just wanted a cuddle."

But as he turned to walk over to the chair to sit down, I got a good look at the little boy's face. Wide and dilated pupils stared back at me. His face was blue. He had not settled. He had stopped breathing. Swinging into emergency mode, I grabbed him from his father's arms and ran with him, shouting to my colleagues to put out the 333 cardiac arrest call.

Laying him down quickly in a cot in the Treatment Room I got a better look at him. Jed was covered in blood. His abdomen had burst and he had experienced catastrophic blood loss. This had led to hypovolemic shock and his heart stopping. I immediately started chest compressions whilst my colleague who had followed me into the Treatment Room used a bag and mask to breathe for him. On a two-year-old much less pressure is needed than with an adult so chest compressions are done with one hand.

"We need blood," I shouted, "quickly."

The crash team consisting of two doctors and a senior nurse rushed in bringing with them the red emergency trolley full of resuscitation equipment and drugs. One doctor quickly got an intravenous line in and started squeezing a bag of fluid into Jed. The other prepared drugs. I continued chest compressions as an auxiliary nurse ran off to the blood bank to get blood. She returned in record time and that too was squeezed into him as quickly as possible.

It was touch and go. A fine line between success and tragedy. Thankfully, we were in time. The fluid brought him back and he started breathing again.

But all I could think about was what if I'd not gone into that room when I did? What if I'd been called away? Or gone to the toilet first? We would very likely have been too late and Jed would have died. That didn't happen and he went on to make a full recovery, but it was the end of my career in Paediatrics. I couldn't cope with the stress of it.

The Senior Sister on the ward, Sister Hartley, radiated kindness and was the epitome of a perfect children's nurse. Having never married, she had dedicated her life to her job. She was calm and twinkly-eyed like a favourite grandma and everyone liked her – both adults and children. It gave me a comforting feeling to know she had been the one to care for Andrea and Mum all those years ago, but talking to her also felt kind of strange, although I'm not sure why.

"I totally understand," she said, when I finally plucked up the courage to tell her I wanted to leave the ward.

"I feel like such a failure, as if I'm letting everyone down."

"You are not letting anyone down," she replied gently. "It's very brave of you to admit it's not working. Hold your head up high and be proud that you tried."

The following week she called me into her office to say that a Staff Nurse working on the surgical unit at Bolton Royal Infirmary wanted to work on Paediatrics. Would I like to swap jobs with her? Again, at the time this was the way things were often done. No application forms or interviews were required. So I swapped with her and my adult nursing career began.

This was also the time when Intensive Care Units were beginning to take off. They were nothing like the ICUs of today that are bristling with technical equipment and computers, and they were nowhere near as big. At Bolton Royal Infirmary, the ICU was a three-bedded bay at the end of a general surgical ward with a curtain pulled across it for privacy. I started working in there and quickly became hooked. The one-to-one nursing suited me perfectly as I loved being able to focus wholly on one patient and do everything for them without having the demands of the rest of the ward pulling on me. The variety of cases ranged from post-surgical complications through to road traffic accidents, cardiac problems and neurological issues. Now, there are specialised units for such things as Neuro and Cardiac but then it was very much a general unit that dealt with everything. I loved the challenge of getting to grips with and learning all about the ventilators and infusion pumps that were used, and the myriad of different drugs needed to treat such conditions required real focus to get to grips with.

It was a good move; the role provided perfect conditions that enabled me to thrive. Of course, by the very nature of Intensive Care, the patients were all very poorly and some of them inevitably passed away. But because they were adults I could cope, although it was still very sad.

Critical Care training courses came thick and fast so as time progressed I became highly skilled and experienced in this newly emerging discipline.

Becoming more senior brought with it more responsibility and therefore more money, and it wasn't long before my thoughts turned to travelling. I still longed to see the world and experience the joy of flying. A few holidays abroad followed but they weren't enough; I wanted more than just to sit on a beach and sunbathe.

Soon, the idea of working in the USA appeared on my radar. Lots of opportunities popped up on the pages of the nursing magazines I bought. They seemed a gift. On offer was sponsorship to travel with everything from a job to accommodation included. They also dangled good salaries and the security of being with a group of other nurses instead of completely alone. And Critical Care experience was very much in demand. As an experienced ICU nurse, the job offers flowed in and I had the luxury of several enticing options to choose from. To sit the Registered Nurse exam – the American equivalent of our Registered General Nurse qualification – you had to go to the States so off I went to Florida. After passing that, a whirlwind of paperwork followed and then I found myself sitting on a 737 bound for Phoenix, Arizona; the location of my new job.

A vast and hot landscape greeted me and I quickly threw myself into life in a large American hospital. There were lots of differences, the main one being the sheer size of the place: the unit I worked on had twenty beds, so more than six times bigger than my previous unit. Everyone was welcoming and friendly, inviting me to their homes for supper and taking me on days out. But it was more difficult than I anticipated and I struggled.

The scale of everything was overwhelming and the hours I was expected to work exhausted me. They had a system very different to the UK whereby if the unit went quiet – like in the middle of the night – you would be 'flexed off' and sent home. I often found myself being sent home at 2 or 3 o'clock in the morning. But if the unit then got busy again, they would call you up and expect you to go back in, even if you had only left an hour ago. This was incredibly tiring to be in and out so much and also meant that to get your contracted hours in you often worked part of every single day without a clear day off. Determined to give it a good shot, I soldiered on for a few months. But by this time I was getting fed up of the difficult working pattern and I was really missing my family.

Reluctantly, I made the decision to come home. Again, it felt as if I had failed, but I tried to reframe it as 'at least I had the courage to give it a go'. I felt that going forward I would be happiest basing myself in England and travelling regularly rather than actually working and living abroad. That seemed like the option that would give me the best of both worlds. But, as I had already found out, one or two holidays a year just wasn't going to cut it.

How could I combine my job with my love of flying and adventure whilst still being based in the UK?

The answer came some time later in the form of a tiny, two-line advert in a nursing magazine:

'Wanted: In-Flight Nurse. Must be Critical Care Trained and Experienced'.

I had never even heard of an In-Flight Nurse and had no idea what one was. But I saw the words Flight' and 'Nurse' and was instantly intrigued.

The advert gave a phone number so I immediately rang to find out more. The job entailed flying all over the World – mostly on commercial flights but sometimes on an air ambulance – to bring people back home to the UK after they had been taken ill or injured abroad. In short, it was my dream job. Excitement raced through me. Within minutes of hanging up the phone, I was preparing my application. It seemed too good to be true, and I didn't expect to get it. They would have hundreds of applicants for such a fabulous job – I had more chance of winning the lottery. But I fired off my application, remembering the old saying, 'You've got to be in it to win it'. If I didn't try I'd never know.

In fact, they had well over two hundred applicants but I was one of the lucky ten who were shortlisted and invited to interview. Nervous, excited, thrilled – I was all of these things. This was my chance to combine my love of caring for people with my love of travelling and adventure. Could I actually get this? Would I be good enough? I was determined to give it my best shot. Interview day arrived – the 6th April. Long before the sun roused itself from slumber, I was dressed and ready to go. Road works and traffic congestion slowed things up as I drove down to Oxford but I had allowed plenty of time. This was one appointment I did not want to be late for.

The repatriation company was housed in a beautiful old converted farm building with extensive grounds. A sweeping gravel drive led up to the front entrance whilst to the back a large terrace overlooked a deer park. It was green, and lush, and so picturesque it looked as if it should belong to The National Trust.

After initial introductions, coffee and biscuits were served outside in the spring sunshine as we all chatted and got to know each other a little. A pretty diverse range of people, we were all from various critical care backgrounds: there was Peter from A&E; Jill from ICU; Jake from Coronary Care. Everyone was smartly dressed and acted calm and professional but underneath I sensed the same simmering mixture of anxiety and excitement that bubbled in me. I plastered a smile on my face but did feel very much out of my depth as every one of them seemed to have such a wealth of experience with qualifications in just about every critical care skill you could think of. I seriously doubted that I could ever be the best of this bunch in order to get the job and my confidence dipped low as we headed inside to get started.

Two role play scenarios saw us acting out various emergency situations and then we were called in one by one for individual interviews. Tom, the doctor who owned the company, was leading the panel along with Fiona who was the In-Flight Nurse Manager. I tried my best to answer their questions calmly and knowledgably but several times my nerves took over, throwing my words out in an incomprehensible babble. Coming out of the room, my mood sank even lower as I was convinced that I had blown it.

After the interviews were finished, Tom gave us the unexpected news that he was actually going to be taking on five of us that day not one. On hearing this, my mood lightened a little as it increased my chances substantially but I still hardly dared to get my hopes up.

"Go to lunch," he said, "and then I'll call you back in when we've made our decision."

This was another bit of good news as we had no idea we were going to be finding out there and then whether we had been successful. I had expected to have to go home and wait for a letter to drop on the mat or a phone call.

Lunch was a spread of sandwiches and cakes back out on the terrace but I don't think any of us did more than pick at the food.

One or two of the lads cracked a few jokes but the tension was so tangible it felt like something you could reach out and twang like a guitar string. It was obvious that every one of us really wanted this job. Sixty minutes crawled by. The wait was excruciating. I watched the deer in the paddock and drank a lot of coffee.

Eventually, Tom called us back in. He would read out the five names of the successful candidates; the other five would then leave. I clutched my handbag tightly on my knee, slapped a smile on my face and waited, hardly daring to breath. Please let my name be called.

First, Tom said Peter's name, then Jill's, then Jake. Just two more names to go. I held my breath. Tom paused, looked straight at me.

And then he said my name.

I didn't hear anything else that was said after that. Nor was I aware of the unsuccessful candidates getting up and leaving. A bubble of disbelief descended on me and the whole room receded into a blur of muted colours and distant sounds. It felt as if I'd entered some kind of third dimension, some world other than the one I normally inhabited. Tom had said my name. It didn't feel real. Had that really just happened? Or was my mind playing a cruel joke on me? And then the room gradually came back into focus. There was laughing and chattering and people congratulating me. Oh my goodness, I had only gone and done it! I was going to be an In-Flight Nurse! My breath rushed out as the tension released, and then another thought occurred to me: this is what it must feel like to win the lottery.

CHAPTER 12

Belize

I am almost certain that within the next thirty seconds I am going to throw up. My stomach is a washing machine, flipping its contents head over heels, sloshing to and fro with a manic-like vengeance. In fact, it feels like I am actually *in* a washing machine. We are dipping and diving above the jungle, skimming the trees so closely it must surely be only a matter of minutes before we crash into them. My mind goes into overdrive imagining the twisted metal, the searing heat, the fact that we are in the middle of nowhere. Would we ever be found if we crashed? And if they did find us how would they get us out? I take a deep breath; give myself a stern talking to. The pilot knows what he is doing. He is trained and experienced, has done this trip many times. It will be fine. My mind is not convinced. The spin cycle gathers pace. I am going to be sick.

When I had first seen the sleek, dark blue helicopter, a familiar sense of excitement tickled my veins. It was standing in the morning sun, gleaming and beautiful, its rotor blades bobbing gently in the breeze. What a magnificent sight. And I was going to get to fly in her.

We were in Belize in Central America, and my patient was Geoff, a research scientist working on a biodiversity project out in the depths of the jungle. Having suffered a bad bout of malaria, he was improving but was still quite unwell so was coming home to the UK for a period of recuperation. I had been asked to go and get him. But until landing in Belize I hadn't realised that

Geoff was still at the research camp in the middle of the jungle. And that it would take a helicopter to reach him. All part of the fun, I thought, as I imagined myself as a female Bear Grylls, taking on the wilderness and having a grand old time whilst doing it.

But that was a very naïve notion and so far, the reality was more abstract terror than fun.

Having never been in a helicopter before I had eagerly strapped myself in and popped on the headset, grinning away at the middle-aged pilot and trying not to look like a slightly demented teenager who has just won a prize at the school disco. He grinned back at me and a prickle of unease crackled through me. He looked 'normal' enough with his close-cropped brown hair and suntanned face, but there was something about him that was triggering my alarm bells; a dangerous edge lurking beneath his benign features and khaki shirt. My Dad had always taught me to trust my instincts but this time I ignored his advice and told myself not to be such a worrier; to get on with being excited at my first helicopter flight. In any case, I didn't have much of a choice as I had a patient to collect and this was the only way to do it.

A few minutes into the flight it became obvious the dangerous edge I'd sensed in 'Tim' was in fact a steak of pure daredevil recklessness. Fast and lose, he started to throw the machine around the sky as if it were a toy, seemingly oblivious to the fact that we were inches from the trees below. Or that I was turning green in the backseat. I fixed my gaze on the back of his neck and hung on for dear life, fighting to keep my breakfast down.

But then very strangely something started to shift within me. My stomach decided it quite liked the spin cycle and my nausea suddenly vanished. Could it possibly be that this was rather thrilling? My fingers still gripped tightly onto the seat but I was surprised to find myself actually beginning to enjoy this crazy ride. Tim glanced over his shoulder at me and flashed a grin.

"Faster?" he mouthed. Against my better judgement I nodded. Faster.

Up, down, left, right. The canopy of trees screamed past beneath us – a blurred mass of green-ness. It felt as if we were totally weightless. Behind me, my brain struggled to catch up with the rest of me. I was light headed and giddy; breathless and grinning. It was electrifying. Was this how the swifts felt when they whooshed across the skies at home? Before I knew it I was shouting for Tim to go faster still. What the heck was I doing? Did I have a death wish? Tim coaxed the whirlybird with his expert hand and just like a racehorse at the end of a race, she gave us everything she had. We truly were flying in every sense of the word, absolutely at the edge of what was possible. Magic.

By the time we landed in a circular clearing at the research camp – amazingly still in one piece - and I clambered out of the helicopter, my legs were jelly and I could barely walk straight. I was laughing like a lunatic, my usual composure having well and truly deserted me. But what a ride! The most thrilling thing I'd ever done. I decided there and then that I liked this crazy bloke named Tim and his ever-so-slightly 'dangerous streak'.

From the clearing, a rough path led me through the trees to the camp mess tent where Geoff was waiting for me. As a research scientist, I had imagined him to be a David Attenborough look alike with a studious face and a gravitas conferred by the important work he was engaged in. In reality, he was a small portly man with thinning hair and wire glasses, sitting at a makeshift table drinking tea and doing a crossword puzzle. Dressed in a baggy beige t-shirt and jeans he looked much older than his forty six years; maybe some of that due to his illness giving him a grey tinge to his face and bags under his eyes. He greeted me with a nod when I introduced myself and then carried on doing his crossword puzzle. It seemed his interest in going home was lukewarm at best.

Unperturbed, I got out my stethoscope and blood pressure machine and began doing my checks. Geoff didn't engage with me but he let me do his blood pressure and oxygen levels. His observations were all satisfactory, and within thirty minutes Tim was winging us back to the airport, thankfully a little more sedately this time as we had the patient on board.

Geoff still didn't say much; he didn't seem to want to talk so I let him be. If he wanted to just relax and conserve his energy then that was fine with me although the thought of the long flight home with a patient who was uncommunicative did fill me with a little unease. Not least because it is difficult to judge how someone is coping with a journey if they don't talk to you.

At the airport he sat staring into the distance for most of the time, seemingly totally disinterested in the hustle and bustle going on around us. When I got coffee for us he gave me a cursory nod of thanks but then slipped back into silence as he sipped his drink.

I was relieved that once airborne on our scheduled flight back to the UK his distant mood gradually started to lift. At first it was just general chit chat about his colleagues at the camp and what their day to day life was like. Then he progressed to tales of jungle encounters with monkeys and spiders and lying awake at night listening for leopards and other large predators. And then he started talking about his work. The research project that had taken him to the jungle three months earlier involved studying different types of plants that were prevalent there. Initially, I listened with fascination as he detailed some of their findings. Unfortunately though the more he talked the more arrogant his tone became. Geoff seemed to have a massive ego that he loved to polish with his words. The conversation involving both of us gradually morphed in to a monologue where Geoff droned on about how wonderful his research was and how he was going to solve all the problems of the world single-handedly. Slowly but steadily I found myself starting to dislike him intensely and wishing he would shut up. A real case of 'be careful what you wish for'.

Of course I still attended to all his needs checking his observations and making sure he was comfortable and had everything he wanted; giving good care was always my first priority whether I liked the patient or not. In practice it very rarely happened that I didn't like a patient but, being only human, it is bound to happen from time to time. Some people will just not be on the same wavelength.

Thankfully Geoff remained medically well during the journey but it is safe to say the flight did its best to wear me down. Waving goodbye to him at Heathrow was definitely the best part of this trip. Apart from my washing machine ride with Tim, of course. Now that was something else!

CHAPTER 13

Sydney

Things were very busy at this point and the trips were coming in thick and fast. But whilst the variety of jobs I was being given was superb, there was one place I was longing to go. Most definitely the top of my wish list, it was the big daddy of them all: Australia.

A rainy Monday morning in October ushered me off to the gym for a swim so when Julie rang I missed the call. She left me a message containing the magic word: Sydney. I immediately rang her back. The phone was engaged. I hung up and tried again. By the third try panic was creeping up on me. Was she in the process of giving the job to someone else because she couldn't get hold of me? I tried again and again, the beep, beep, beep taunting me down the line. Eventually, after what seemed like a hundred tries, she picked up. And my dream trip was gifted to me. I was going to Australia.

Four days later, I set off for Heathrow on my biggest adventure yet. Heading to Sydney via Singapore with Singapore Airlines, I settled in for the long trip, enjoying all the paraphernalia that comes with flying long haul. To this day, my brother Andrew thinks I'm mad to enjoy flying on commercial aircraft and can see no reason what-so-ever to enjoy an airport. Admittedly, as already said, Heathrow isn't my favourite but I still love the spectacle of it. And the knowing that when you touch down again, you will be on the other side of the world. Safe to say, Andrew hasn't inherited Dad's love of planes and flying the way I have!

Wining and dining us, the cabin crew, dressed in their beautiful blue sarong kebayas, took superb care of us. I still marvel at how they look so calm, poised and elegant even though they are running up and down the aircraft non-stop. On such a long flight – about thirteen hours to Singapore – there are two crew teams so they can take breaks. Reassuring to know when you are in the air for so long that there are several pilots on board.

I read, watched a couple of films, had a sleep – all the usual things you do on a long haul flight. But, even for someone like me who loves flying, there is no denying that London to Singapore is an extremely long flight that challenges you physically. Early on I learned to always book an aisle seat whenever I could so that I could have more space and be able to get up and move around frequently. Flying so many miles so often I knew I was at increased risk of a Deep Vein Thrombosis – a potentially life threatening blood clot in the legs caused by sitting for long periods of time – so I was always careful to move as much as I could and to drink plenty of water to prevent dehydration causing thickening of the blood. Flying has a dehydrating effect on the body so this is super important.

Many thousands of miles later, the plane touched down safely in Singapore. With six hours to wait before my connection to Sydney, I set off to explore Changi International Airport. And what a beautiful airport. Serene Koi Carp pools provided a tranquil spot to relax away from the hustle and bustle of the main concourse. Then I was delighted to find there was also a butterfly house. Considering it is such a busy international airport full of shops and people, the peaceful oasis in the middle of it all was a surprise and a pleasure. Being stiff from the flight I wanted to have a good walk to stretch my legs so I moved on and happily trotted around the shops buying one or two pretty little trinkets to take home. The Singapore Lion – half lion, half fish - intrigued me. Apparently the fishy lower half comes from the origins of Singapore as a fishing village whilst the lion's head comes from the word Singapura – the original name for Singapore - literally meaning Lion City in Malay. At the time I had a thing for collecting key rings, and there were many Singapore Lions in every colour imaginable catching my eye as I wondered around, so yet another one was added to my growing collection.

It's a strange fact of travelling that although you're often sat for long periods of time doing nothing to get dirty, you always feel grubby. You are showered, hair done, clothes freshly ironed when you set off but before long the wrinkly, grubby feeling takes hold. Freshening up in an aircraft toilet is better than nothing but not particularly effective or enjoyable. Wet wipes are the same – better than nothing but not fantastic. Changi has considered this and thoughtfully provided shiny new shower and toilet facilities that wouldn't be out of place in a five star hotel. They are absolutely gorgeous with sumptuous decoration and state of the art facilities. With time still to kill I washed and changed, instantly feeling better and getting my 'second wind'.

The biggest chunk of the trip – thirteen hours – was done, just seven more to go aboard a majestic Boeing 747. Her white livery with bluebird tail sparkled in the sunshine as I watched the ground crew loading her up through the windows. Gigantic, like no other plane I'd ever been on, I marvelled that something so big could actually get off the ground. On later trips I would fly the Airbus 380 which is even bigger. What fantastic feats of engineering these planes are – real marvels of modern technology and innovation. And, of course, the 747 has now been decommissioned so I feel really lucky to have had the pleasure of flying on her.

But get off the ground we did, and soon we were airborne on the last leg of the trip. Some hours later the pilot announced, "Ladies and gentlemen, we are now flying over Australia." We've made good time I thought, nearly there; only to then have the sheer enormity of Australia make itself known. We were over the West Coast and there was still hours to go to get to Sydney on the East Coast. Of course, I knew it was a vast continent, but it was still an eye-opener to actually experience it. The other thing that I had become acutely aware of as we rounded the globe was what an awfully long way away from home Australia actually is. You know the numbers of how many thousands of miles away the continent lies from the UK but it's only when you are actually flying for hours and hours, getting further and further away, that the reality of it sinks in. I really was on the other side of the world – the furthest I would ever be from home. And my family. And everything that made up the minutia of my life. From nowhere a sudden stab of loneliness took me by surprise. I had no idea why – I was only here for a few days and then would be heading back to everything I knew and loved. What reason did I have to be lonely? Was this not my grandest adventure yet? Sometimes, I suppose, there is no rhyme or reason - feelings are just feelings. You sit with them and experience them, and then you let them go.

By the time we landed the feeling had passed and I felt better. Clearing customs, I checked my watch - 7am. Tiredness had soaked into my bones after the 24 hour journey but a surge of adrenaline as I stepped out into the Sydney sunshine boosted me on. This was it. I was here. In Australia.

Julie had booked me into a hotel at Darling Harbour, a vibrant waterfront area of the city, so I jumped in a waiting taxi. It was too early to check in but I hoped they would let me leave my bag so that I could head out for some sightseeing without carting it around with me. My trusty purple rucksack was still my bag of choice but this trip it was crammed to the gills with extra clothes as well as my medical equipment.

With only 24 hours until I collected my patient, sightseeing time was severely limited so after the hotel I powered on through the tiredness and set off to see as much as I could. Top of my list of things to see was The Opera House. It didn't disappoint. As I walked towards Circular Quay and got my first glimpse of those iconic sails gleaming in the morning sun, I actually got a lump in my throat and thought I might cry! What a totally unexpected reaction. I guess it spoke volumes about how much visiting this stunning place meant to me. In a way it made me feel that if I could come here and do this on my own, then I could do anything. I sat for a long time on the grass by the harbour listening to the street artists that lined the Quay.

Steel drums and digeridoos played alongside each other whilst the green and yellow Manley Ferries sprinted backwards and forwards across the water. And all the while, The Opera House presided over it all like a priceless pearl at the centre of an oyster.

I set off to walk around it, taking my time and savouring every moment. I tried to remember each and every detail so that I'd be able to bring the image to life at will: the smooth cream tiles, the cascading steps, the huge windows. A flotilla of tiny sailing boats, white against the deep blue water, was escorting a cruise ship into the harbour. The Captain hooted the horn as it passed the Opera House and I joined the crowds waving back to the cheering passengers on deck. What a spectacular moment that must have been for them – sailing into Sydney Harbour at the end of a long voyage and being greeted by the jewel in Australia's crown. It was probably the highlight of their holiday.

And there was no doubt in my mind that I wanted to return here on holiday myself. All of the places I've been to have been interesting; some have been more enjoyable than others. But Sydney and The Opera House had that something extra. That ethereal, indefinable ingredient that dances around at the edge of your emotions. You feel the shiver, the connection, the thrill. It was something I'd never experienced before. And I knew I wanted more.

But for now, sadly, my time had run out. I needed to head back to my hotel to eat and sleep before picking up my patient the next day.

"There's a message for you," the receptionist said as I checked in. She handed me a note asking me to phone Julie at the office. Working out the time difference, I realised I'd have to wait a couple of hours before I could ring her as it was the early hours of the morning back in the UK. I went to eat, wondering what she wanted me for and hoping it wasn't bad news.

"Your patient has had a pulmonary embolism so he's not fit to fly," she said when I managed to get through some time later. "You had already left when we found out."

"Oh no, what a shame, poor man," I replied. "So am I heading back tomorrow?"

"Well, we've been looking at options and we think it will be cheaper to let you wait there for him rather than to fly you home and then back again in a few days. What do you think? Would that be ok with you?"

I felt like Maggie, the Scottish lady in Mallorca, and almost did a little dance. Would that be ok? Most certainly it would!

"I'll book you into the hotel for another few days," Julie went on. "He's doing ok so they are estimating he'll be fit to fly in four or five days. Just buy whatever you need, keep your receipts and we'll cover it."

This was definitely a 'pinch me' moment that I couldn't quite believe was really happening. I was to ring the hospital daily to see how my patient, Bill, was but other than that the next few days were mine. I could do whatever I liked, was booked into a nice four star hotel, and had an expense account to pay for meals and essentials. On top of that I would get paid my normal daily rate of pay for every day that I was away so would also get a nice pay packet when I got home. Things like this don't happen to me, I thought, but then I smiled to myself – yes, they do! The only downside was that I was on my own so had no one to share it with. But I have travelled and holidayed alone on many occasions so it wasn't really an issue. Of course, I was sad Bill had had a setback but he was doing okay so hopefully that's all it would be and in four to five days' time he would be fit to travel home.

Just to mention at this point that although we always had our expenses covered, I never abused the system. I would always eat in cheap and cheerful places, drank barely any alcohol and, in cases like this, would only buy absolute essentials. Any treats, trips etc. I always paid for out of my own money. I've no doubt that some did take advantage but I never did. I considered I was extremely lucky to be doing what I was doing and that was enough for me.

Four days later, Sydney waved me on my way with many special memories. The highlight was a whale watching trip out into the harbour where our boat was treated to a visit by two orca.

It was impossible not to be enthralled by their presence as their tails slapped the water and they circled around our boat happily putting on a display that lasted nearly twenty minutes. Strange to think what skilful predators they are and how aggressive they can be; it seemed really at odds with how beautiful and graceful they were.

Climbing the Harbour Bridge created more thrills and also introduced me to Edith. Edith was a remarkable woman. Six weeks into a solo trip around Australia, she had spent time in the bush, visited the kangaroos in Alice Springs and sailed around the Great Barrier Reef. Edith also climbed the bridge with us. And the most remarkable part? She was eighty-six years old! What a lady.

And so it was time to leave. Cities have never really been my thing, always preferring the wide open spaces of the countryside, but Sydney infused every cell in my body with wonder. She delighted me at every turn. I vowed to return on holiday and delve deeper into her colour and vibrancy. But for now my patient had been passed as fit to fly, so it was time to go and get him home to his family.

Bill was in a hospital in a small, rural town to the north of Sydney so I boarded a sleek silver train that was shimmering in the forty-degree heat. Suburbs flashed by in a whirl of colour to gradually be replaced by large expanses of dusty nothingness. Eventually, the train rumbled up to my stop and after disembarking I watched it gather pace again heading off towards the hazy horizon. I was the only person to leave the train.

As usual, I made my way out of the station, which in this case was actually just a platform sheltered by a tin roof, and looked for a taxi to take me to the hospital. But there were no taxis. In fact there were no people. It suddenly dawned on me there was no anything. I did a slow 360 degree turn surveying my surroundings. An arrow-straight road stood deserted by the platform but other than that it was just empty red desert as far as the eye could see in every direction. It was like something out of The Thornbirds – a classic Australian film I had seen years before.

It's easy to let your imagination run wild when you find yourself stranded in the middle of nowhere. Visions of still being here three days later, dying a horrible death shrivelled in the baking sun, crowded into my head. I rolled my eyes and told myself to get a grip. The town must be close, maybe I could walk; the trouble was I had no idea which direction to go in as there were absolutely no landmarks at all. I was perching by the roadside trying to figure out my next move when thankfully a white four-wheel-drive appeared spewing out a large cloud of red dust in its wake as it slid to a halt beside me.

"You ok, luv?" the driver asked, popping a tanned face with crinkly blue eyes out of the car window. Around thirty-ish, dressed all in khaki with a thick Australian accent, he made me feel as if I'd hopped out of The Thornbirds and in to Crocodile Dundee. I half expected a digeridoo soundtrack to start playing and him to ask me if I wanted to go walkabout. But I was never the less very pleased to see him.

"I'm looking for a taxi or a bus," I said. "Do you know if there's any due?"

He laughed good naturedly. "Not today, luv. I think the next bus is tomorrow afternoon. You going to the hospital by any chance?"

"Yes," I replied warily. "How did you know?"

"Not much else here, luv. Jump in, I'll take you."

"Are you sure?" I asked, once again wondering if I was going to be murdered and never seen again.

He flashed a big grin. "Sure, no worries, jump in. It's only down the road."

I seriously doubted that it was 'only down the road' as there was literally nothing to see in any direction. But he was right. I'd no sooner settled into the passenger seat than we were heading into a dip where the town suddenly appeared like a mirage in front of me. I say 'town' but it was really just a handful of local shops and a pub lining one street with a few people and stray dogs going slowly about their business.

"The hospital's there," said my saviour pointing to the end of the street. "Just behind the post office."

Grateful to have arrived safely, and to not be dying by the side of the road, I shook the proffered hand.

"The name's Chris," he said. "I own a farm up the road. Give me a call if you need anything."

"Thank you, Chris, I will," I replied. "Do you have a number?"

"Just ask Betty on the desk to call me, she's my Mum."

"Aahh, right," I said, the penny dropping. "So is that maybe how you knew I was heading to the hospital?"

"You got me," he laughed. "She told me they were expecting a nurse from England and you just kinda looked like 'a nurse from England'."

Laughing myself, I thanked him again and waved as he headed off down the street, honking his horn and creating a cloud of red dust that enveloped me. I wondered how Bill came to be in such a tiny, off- the-beaten-track kind of place; it didn't seem like somewhere you would head to on your holidays.

A wonderful blast of air conditioned coolness drew me into the hospital and Betty turned out to be just as friendly as her son. Within minutes she had bustled out from behind her desk, her glasses bobbing on her chest at the end of a gold chain, and shown me where I could freshen up. I was mightily hot and bedraggled by this point, not to mention covered in red dust. She also provided me with a bottle of ice cold water and directions to Bill's ward. Making my way along the corridors it struck me how light and spacious the hospital was. After seeing the small, rural town, I was expecting an old fashioned cottage-style hospital but instead found gleaming chrome and light filled walk ways. I was learning that my expectations were often wide of the mark.

A quick push on the bell by the ward door was answered by a smiling nurse in white scrubs. Betty had rung ahead so I was expected and welcomed and after quick introductions she showed me to Bill's room. A billowing mass of pillows cocooned him and their stark whiteness made him look thin and pale, but he was settled and comfortable, his eyes closed and his breathing steady as he slept. I slipped quietly in trying not to disturb him but the click of the door closing behind me caused his eyes to flicker open. I smiled.

"Hi," I said. "I'm Wendy, the nurse from the UK. I'm here to take you home."

My words cleared his sleepy expression and he returned my smile.

Throughout my career as an In-Flight Nurse I was always greeted with relief and happiness. It didn't matter how good the hospital was or how kind and caring the staff were, the patients were at a low point in a foreign country and they couldn't wait to get home to the safety and familiarity of family and loved ones. Often times they were alone so the relief of having someone with them, organising and doing whatever was necessary to get them safely home, was palpable. Sometimes there was also a language barrier to cope with so they would not really know what was going on. Having someone to explain things to them and sort everything out for their journey home lifted a huge weight off their shoulders and you could often see them visibly relax the minute they realised who I was. And from my point of view it was very uplifting and rewarding to always have people pleased to see me. No matter how hard the journey or what problems cropped up it was always worth it.

Bill had been on holiday when he had sadly been involved in a serious accident. Unfortunately this had resulted in him having to have his right leg amputated below the knee. Shocked and struggling to cope with this, his recovery had been slower than expected. To compound his problems a blood clot had then lodged in his lung – the pulmonary embolism that had delayed our departure. As a retirement treat – he was sixty six with forty years as a plumber under his belt – he had been on a dream holiday with his wife touring around Australia in a campervan. Just one week into their six week adventure, the van had suffered a tyre blow out when they were travelling at sixty miles per hour. Careering into a ditch, the van had rolled over. Sally, Bill's wife had fortunately suffered just cuts and bruises but Bill had been trapped, his leg crushed under the weight of the steering column. Instead of going home with fabulous memories of their once-in-a-life-time trip, he was now going home minus a leg.

Sally had already flown on ahead so it was just going to be Bill and me. Emirates were flying us as far as Dubai. Once there we would meet up with another nurse who would take over Bill's care for the Dubai to Heathrow part of the journey. I was glad about this having realised on the way out just what a long and tiring trip it was. Looking after a patient for the whole twenty-four-hour journey would have been exhausting and potentially very unsafe. I was still doing the longest part of the trip though so had made sure to be well rested and prepared.

I busied around packing up Bill's things ready to leave whilst chatting away to him asking him about his wife and family. Despite his shrunken appearance and the weary edge that rimmed his eyes, he happily told me all about his grown up daughters in a rich, deep Yorkshire accent that gave a clue about the strong, fit man he normally was. Used to always being busy and on the go running his own business, the enforced bed rest had dragged him down but now that he was going home he was quite animated and cheerful. A steady and strong pulse coupled with a surprisingly healthy blood pressure reading of 130/80 confirmed he was fit to fly. The nurse in charge of the ward handed over to me telling me what care Bill had received and what medication he was on. Co-codamol tablets were signed out to me for when he needed pain relief and his paperwork was put in an envelope ready to go. He didn't currently need oxygen but it was booked for the flight as a precaution. An aircraft cabin has less circulating oxygen available so sometimes a patient who is fine at ground level will become hypoxic – oxygen depleted – at altitude and will therefore need support. Once airborne you are stuck so everything you might need is booked and taken to try and ensure you have everything you could possibly need. This is even more important when it is such a long flight.

Bill had a urine catheter so I emptied the bag and fastened it securely with Velcro straps to his remaining leg. Lastly, I helped him change out of his pyjamas and into track suit pants and a t-shirt. Checking his stump as I did so, the dressing was clean and dry with no evidence of swelling or infection. Bill avoided looking at it – a common reaction when suffering a new amputation. It would take a while for him to adjust and come to terms with his altered body image. Having had a shave that morning, all that was left to do was comb his hair and help him put on his watch.

"Ready for off?" I asked.

"Ready," he said. "I feel better already. Strange how just combing your hair and putting on your watch can make you feel more normal again."

The staff lined the corridor as we headed out, their claps and cheers waving us off. It seemed they had developed a soft spot for the gentle Yorkshire man and were thrilled he was now well enough to go home. We were on our way. Only ten thousand miles to go.

Our ambulance made good time to the airport and Bill remained relaxed and happy. He needed to have his amputated leg elevated for the journey home so we were travelling in Business Class with reclining seats and more space. The Business Class lounge with floor to ceiling windows provided us with a great view of the aircraft as we waited to board.

As usual, we were boarded first which made it easier to get Bill comfortable whilst the cabin was empty. I wrapped him up warmly in blankets and padded his leg with pillows whilst a flight attendant brought him orange juice to drink. At this point he still seemed fine with his observations all remaining stable, although he had gone a bit quieter. I presumed he was just tired with all the excitement and would probably fall asleep pretty quickly once we were airborne. It was a huge undertaking for anyone going from weeks in a hospital bed to a ten thousand mile journey home.

The other passengers boarded - mostly business people in suits and carrying laptop bags – and the cabin hummed with quiet conversation and the tapping of computer keys.

When working, I didn't wear a uniform, just jeans and a blue polo shirt with a name badge. As such, when I was travelling with a seated patient, I think the other passengers thought I was a relative rather than a nurse. This could sometimes lead to some strange looks and occasionally the odd comment about my 'Mum' or 'Dad'.

After take-off we were served a beautifully cooked meal that Bill ate and enjoyed then the cabin crew dimmed the lights so we could rest. Unexpectedly this seemed to upset Bill. He started to fidget, pulling at his blankets and shifting around in his seat as if he were uncomfortable. I talked quietly to him trying to find out what was bothering him and to soothe him but he gradually became more restless and unsettled. I thought maybe the lower oxygen levels in the cabin air were affecting him so I started him on oxygen via nasal cannula. He wouldn't let me put the pulse oximeter on his finger so I didn't know what his actual oxygen saturation was but I knew it would do no harm and hoped it would help. It didn't. Over the next half hour his agitation increased then progressed to confusion. He didn't know who I was or where he was. I persuaded him to take some of his pain killers in case he was in pain but again this had no effect. Then he began throwing off his blankets and trying to pull his urine catheter out. As talked about with Ralph earlier, this is not good. It can cause serious trauma to the patient as the catheter has a balloon on the end that is inflated with water and sits in the bladder to stop the tube falling out. Pulling it out with the balloon fully inflated can rip the patient's urethra. There can also be problems if they are consequently unable to urinate.

By this time, the other passengers who were trying to sleep started to get very annoyed with us for disturbing them. One man very loudly told me to please, "Shut your father up!" The lack of compassion appalled me as it was obvious that Bill was poorly and not just causing problems for the fun of it. I glared pointedly at the man but didn't bother to answer him. Very sad that he couldn't show a little kindness and empathy: what if Bill had been his father? I'm sure he wouldn't have wanted someone telling him to shut up.

In contrast, the purser in the cabin, a middle-aged gentleman named Mo, came over to see if he could assist in any way. He helped me to adjust Bill's position and brought more pillows to try and make him more comfortable. All the while he was talking to Bill in a soft, gentle voice and his smile was kind and genuine.

Eventually, it was one of Maggie's 'wee cups of tea' that did the trick; a cup of Earl Grey with a little whiskey in it. (Although not as much whiskey as Maggie used to have in hers!) Slowly, he started to calm down as the drink soothed him. A few minutes later his eyes began to close and his chin dipped to his chest as he fell asleep. Mo offered to sit with Bill whilst I used the bathroom and then he made me a hot coffee as my last one had gone untouched – a small kindness that was much appreciated.

Bill slept peacefully for an hour and I was able to relax a bit. The cabin was dark and quiet; the only sounds those of the thrumming engines.

And then all of a sudden Bill shot forward out of his seat and lunged head first towards the galley. I gasped, completely caught off guard. Grabbed for him. Missed. His good leg propelling him at record speed like a sprinter off the blocks. And then he was falling. Crashing towards the floor. His head on course to smash into the wall. I launched myself up to try and stop him but I knew I was too late. But then miraculously Mo was there. Coming out of the galley. Catching him. Breaking his fall and lowering him to the floor.

Instantly I was on my knees at Bill's side, checking him over, looking for injuries. He was shaken up, dazed and muttering, but amazingly unhurt. Mo and I managed to lift him back into his seat and strap him in. I thanked Mo profusely as without his quick reaction it could have been a very different outcome. He just smiled shyly and said it was luck. No doubt there was an element of luck with the timing but there was also his willingness to get involved and to help, something he didn't have to do. And he was the only one that did – everyone else just watched.

The fall seemed to have taken the wind out of Bill's sails, and although he did continue to be disorientated, he calmed down and thankfully stopped trying to pull his catheter out. He also tolerated the oxygen which I had increased to 100%. It was obvious he was not as well as when we had left Australia but his vital signs remained satisfactory so my main goal was still to get him through the flight and home. I would ring Tom at the office when we reached Dubai. An ambulance was already arranged to meet us at Heathrow as Bill was being admitted to St George's but I wanted to get Tom's advice and fill him in on how Bill was.

By the time we reached Dubai my energy was running low. Watching Bill every second to ensure he didn't hurt himself, and trying to keep him comfortable and settled, was very full on. On a number of occasions he tried to get up again, albeit half-heartedly, and continued to fidget and mutter to himself. No opportunity to have a rest had arisen; I was tired and fighting hard to stay patient and professional. I was very much looking forward to meeting up with my relief nurse, Emma, and to her taking over Bill's care so I could have a break.

We had to change aircraft in Dubai and it had been arranged that we would meet Emma at the departure gate of our Heathrow bound flight. The two hour layover provided an opportunity to take Bill to the toilet and check and empty his catheter out. I also checked his wound dressing and gave him a wash to freshen him up. He was calmer at ground level but still mixed up and not himself, watching my every move as if he suspected I was not who I said I was.

We went to meet Emma but there was no sign of her. Eventually the airport staff came to board us and Emma still hadn't arrived. As we settled in our seats, the cabin manager, Assam, brought me a message: Emma's outbound flight had been delayed so she wouldn't arrive in time. I have to confess, I was gutted. Exhaustion threatened to make me cry. There was still another long flight ahead of us.

One positive thing was that my conversation with Tom had been good. It was reassuring to talk to him and tell him how

Bill had been. He agreed that as Bill's observations were stable we could carry on to London, continuing to give oxygen, regular pain relief and extra fluids as I had been doing. He suspected that Bill had an infection brewing somewhere; possibly a urine infection as they are quite common in catheterized patients. He said he would meet us at Heathrow to check Bill over before we headed to St George's.

But there was the little matter of another eight or so hours in the air to get through first. I metaphorically pulled up my big-girl pants, smiled at Assam and asked for more coffee.

But this trip wasn't done with us yet. It had one more thing up its sleeve to throw at us: a raging storm. The turbulence hit us about two hours into the flight and it threw our ginormous Airbus around in the sky like a child's toy. Up and down we lurched, all service stopped and everyone belted into their seats. It thumped luggage around in the overhead bins and threw drinks down the front of people's shirts. Lightning flashed outside the windows like a dragon spitting fire at us. Further down the plane a group of Arab ladies started wailing and praying. As a frequent flier I have experienced lots of turbulence but this was a pretty spectacular example. For the most part Bill just held my hand and sat staring straight ahead but at one point he did decide he'd had enough and tried to throw himself towards the door. I was very grateful he wasn't a big man or I may have struggled to keep him in his seat – even so I was virtually sitting on top of him to keep him safe.

I was also grateful for Assam. His calm manner made him a perfect cabin manager. Once we were through the storm he moved steadily around reassuring everyone and providing drinks and snacks. I needed to keep Bill well hydrated if, as we suspected, the cause of his confusion was that he had a urine infection brewing. Extra fluids would flush his kidneys and catheter, helping to mitigate the problem until we could get him loaded up with antibiotics. I had a word with Assam. He happily agreed to keep the tea coming and after the turbulence settled, Bill was the first person to get a drink. In fact, after my experience with both Mo on our earlier flight and now Assam, I could honestly say I was very impressed with Emirates' choice and training of staff as they were both superb – a real credit to the airline. And I have not been paid to say that!

The remainder of the flight thankfully passed without incident. Bill slept for most of the time, his hand firmly gripping mine. I felt really sorry for him. Seemingly such an intelligent, smart man reduced to a shell of his former self in just a few weeks. I really hoped he would manage to get some semblance of his previous life back.

I breathed a massive sigh of relief as we landed then taxied towards our gate: we'd made it. Two paramedics came on board to get Bill off. True to his word, Tom was waiting for us in the ambulance out on the tarmac. He checked Bill over and agreed with our earlier suspicions that his problem was likely an infection. He cleared us to carry on to St George's as planned.

At the hospital, further tests revealed that Bill did in fact have a urine infection. This sounds like quite a minor illness but it can cause a significant problem for older people with the main complication being the confusion it causes. It had been unfortunate that he had started to be affected by it just as we were flying home; very likely, the journey exacerbated the problem. But it was a relief to find that the cause of Bill's deterioration was something that was easily treated with antibiotics and fluids and I knew from previous experience that he should pick up quite quickly.

He did indeed pick up quickly and went on to make a very good recovery. A prosthetic leg was custom made for him and after a few months of rehabilitation he was walking again and able to enjoy his retirement. Sally, his wife, sent me a beautiful thank you card with a photo of Bill attached. He had put weight back on, was happy and smiling, and I was thrilled to see he'd done so well. Touchingly, she also included a hand written note from Bill apologizing for being a 'nuisance' on the flight. Much of what happened on the journey home had been swallowed by his confusion but he did remember trying to 'leg it' multiple times and 'grumbling like a grumpy old b****d' when I wouldn't let him. I smiled at his turn of phrase – spoken like a true Yorkshireman. He also said they were planning another trip Down Under – although there was no camper van involved this time! I so hope things went better for them this time round and they got the trip of a lifetime they deserved.

CHAPTER 14

Greece

The minute hand on the departure gate clock swept steadily around the large white face as if taunting me. It had no regard for the knot of unease that was mushrooming in my stomach. Time was passing and that was that. 'Not my problem,' it seemed to say.

In five minutes and thirty seconds it would be exactly four hours since I had last seen my patient. My severely injured, totally helpless, seventeen-year-old patient. The unease I felt was rapidly racing towards serious worry. I took a couple of long, deep breaths. Please let him be okay I muttered to myself as I watched that damn minute hand.

Alex had been enjoying a week's holiday with his parents, Sarah and Don, in Greece. I use the word 'enjoying' in a somewhat limited way as he had actually confessed to me that he hadn't really been enjoying himself much at all. Endless traipsing around old buildings and shops wasn't really his 'thing' but he had been enjoying the hotel pool which had helped to make the holiday a little more bearable.

What he had found decidedly unbearable was the heat. The end of May temperatures on the island had regularly been hitting the mid-thirties. Hot and sticky and humid. Ultimately this led Alex into a situation that very nearly cost him his life.

The third night of the holiday he had been tossing and turning in bed, unable to sleep because he was so hot. Rickety air conditioning battled valiantly against the sweltering heat trapped in his room, but it was failing miserably. Without giving it a second thought, he had done what many of us would do: headed outside for a few minutes to get some fresh air.

Finding a peaceful, quiet terrace, he sat on a step to relax for a few minutes. It was around one am so no one else was about and Alex was pleased to feel a cooling breeze wafting in over the water. The hotel stood overlooking a small bay ringed with rocks and shingle whilst an ink-black sky flickered with stars that seemed to draw his gaze towards them as if magnetized. He allowed his eyes to trace the constellations and idly wondered what it would be like to be an astronaut. He was studying Sports Science at college but had always been fascinated with space. I suspect most little boys at one point or another want to be an astronaut, and Alex had been no different, but even though he had outgrown that particular career choice, his love of space remained.

The gentle sounds of the sea whispering against the rocks combined with the cooling breeze soothed his flushed and sweaty face and lulled Alex into a deep state of relaxation. He felt his eyes beginning to close. Not wanting to go back to the hot, stuffy room, he shuffled back to lean on the wall behind him and have a doze.

At least he thought it was a wall. In the dark, with tiredness clouding his mind, he hadn't taken much notice, being more focussed on catching the breeze and getting some relief from the unrelenting heat. But it wasn't a wall. What it was in fact was a door and when Alex leaned back on it, it gave way. And then he was falling. Flailing around frantically for something to grab onto. Anything to stop his fall. But there was nothing. Just rough concrete walls grazing his fingers. Clouds of dust. Stale air. Heat.

The door smashed shut above him. Then he hit the floor. Hard. And that too was concrete. Alex had fallen thirty feet down an old rubbish chute that was no longer in use. He recalled a few moments of nothingness. Of being in a kind of limbo. He knew he must be seriously hurt but felt no pain; nothing. Did it mean he was paralysed? Had he broken his back and all feeling was gone forever? Pain would have reassured him that he was in fact still alive.

But, as the saying goes, 'Be careful what you wish for'. Because then the pain did hit. Almighty great bullets of it, ricocheting up his spine into his chest and arms. The barrage fired the breath from his lungs leaving him gasping, suffocating in a quagmire of agony. When he tried to breathe more bullets blasted into him like machine gun fire. Then his legs began screaming.

Panic surged within him like an unstoppable monster eager to join in the carnage. But amazingly for someone so young he managed to fight it off. A keen rugby player, Alex had suffered several incidents on the pitch where he had had to battle his way through the pain of injury. Instinctively he took himself to that place of mental strength and imagined his coach, Jeff, talking to him. 'Slowly, Alex, slowly. Count to five. Take gentle breaths. Come on, let's count together. One, two, three, four, five.'

Still the monster raged. But after a few minutes Alex managed to beat it down. His breathing became a little easier. His heart rate slowed by a few beats per minute. He continued to focus, to count slowly to five, again and again. In and out. "That's it," said Jeff. "Keep going. You're doing well. It's going to be alright."

Once his breathing settled, Alex was able to start gathering his thoughts. His eyes flitted around trying to work out where he was. He was lying flat on his back surrounded by what looked like bags of rubbish. In near total darkness, he had no idea how far he'd fallen or whether there was any way out. He doubted he could move anyway even if there was a way out. And in any case, he knew not to move as his back could be broken. The best thing to do he reasoned was to shout for help. It took three attempts before he could summon up enough breath to call out. When he did, the pain in his chest shot off the scale. An involuntary scream escaped his lips. 'Breathe,' said Jeff. 'Breathe. Come on, you can do it. One, two, three, four, five.'

Unfortunately for Alex, as it was the middle of the night, there was no one about to hear him. His parents were fast asleep in bed and didn't even know he'd left his room so no one missed him. He shouted as loud as he could, over and over again, until his throat seized up and his shouts became merely croaks. And then realisation washed over him. He was wasting his time. No one could hear him. But he didn't know what else to do.

He started to think that maybe he would actually die there that night. But then what if he didn't die? Thoughts of being paralysed smashed into him along with anger at himself for not watching more carefully what he was doing. Shock started shaking him and he lay there in the dark feeling hot tears coursing down his cheeks. He hadn't cried since being a small child and he felt so ashamed of himself. His Dad wouldn't cry.

Alex had no idea how much time passed. He drifted in and out of consciousness. He was so cold. How could he be so cold when the heat had been sweltering? Where was he? Was it breakfast time yet? Are you there, Jeff? What's happening?

After what seemed like an eternity daylight began to creep around the edges of the door Alex had fallen through. Voices drifted down in the dust as the hotel cleaning staff began to arrive and start work. 'Alex, wake up!' said Jeff. 'There's someone there. Come on, wake up!' Barely conscious by this stage, Alex just about managed to open his eyes and focus on the sounds above him. 'Come on, Alex, shout, you have to shout!' A sandpaper mouth coated in dust strangled his words. He tried again and again. "Help me, please! Help me!" His voice was hoarse and raspy, but it was there. He was shouting. Louder and louder, more desperate with every try. Eventually he was screaming at the top of his lungs as his mind finally surrendered to the panic monster. Mercifully, it worked: one of the staff heard him. A minute or two went by as they searched for the voice they could hear, and then the door creaked open flooding the chute with early morning sunlight. Alex saw a face peering down at him. Heard someone say, "Oh, my goodness, there's someone down there!" Then the lethal combination of pain and shock overtook him, his vision greyed over and he fell off the cliff into unconsciousness.

Within minutes of the alarm being raised fire crews and an ambulance arrived. But there was a major problem. The old rubbish chute ended in an underground basement which was no longer used. It had been bricked up many years previously. There was no way to get to Alex other than down the chute. This meant valuable time was lost as the fire crews had to rig up climbing equipment in order to be able to get down to him. One fire officer said later that he thought Alex had died. Eventually a fire man was lowered down to him. He strapped an oxygen mask to Alex's face and gave him morphine then a stretcher was lowered down. Carefully Alex was manoeuvred onto it and then he was winched up with a fire man by his side steadying the ascent.

By this time word had spread around the hotel and Sarah and Don had realised Alex was not in his room. They raced around to the terrace just as the stretcher appeared above ground. Sarah was beside herself and clung anxiously onto Don's hand as they pushed their way forward. When she saw her son she nearly fainted. It was 7am – Alex had been lying in the basement for nearly six hours. Concrete dust coated his body making him look so ghostly that Sarah thought he was dying. The oxygen mask covered most of his face and his arms were lying at odd angles on his chest, obviously badly broken. Strapped to a spinal board, blood was oozing from his head and running down his cheek. Pushing past the firemen, Sarah frantically called Alex's name. She desperately tried to wipe the blood from his face with a tissue until Don gently pulled her back.

"Come on, luv, we have to let them get him to the hospital."

Sarah allowed herself to be pulled back. The stretcher with Alex strapped to it disappeared in to the back of the waiting ambulance. She felt a sob escape her lips. Would that be the last time they saw their son alive? She turned to Don. Saw tears in his eyes too. It was to be a very long and arduous day for them both.

After the blue light dash to the hospital, hours passed by with excruciating slowness as the doctors attempted to stabilise Alex. He was ventilated and scanned, dripped and given life-saving drugs. And then Sarah and Don were given the news that their son had broken nearly every bone in his body: both arms, both legs, several spinal vertebra, 4 ribs, and a hairline fracture to his skull. Sarah recalled the moment she heard the words, 'several spinal vertebra'.

"I felt bile rising in my throat," she told me. "I just couldn't contemplate that my fit, rugby-playing seventeen-year-old son might end up in a wheelchair for the rest of his life."

After a shocked pause it was Don who asked the doctor the question, "Will he be paralysed?"

And then amazingly, the sombre, grey-haired man smiled. "That is the good news today," he said. "There appears to be no damage to his spinal cord. I think, with a lot of care and rehabilitation, that your son will make a good recovery."

Being young and fit meant Alex coped well with the emergency surgery he needed to fix both his legs. A brace supported his back whilst the vertebrae healed and both arms were placed in plaster casts. The hairline fracture to his skull would heal itself as would his ribs – luckily they hadn't punctured his lungs. All in all, although it didn't seem it at the time, he was a very lucky young man.

Progress was steady and it was soon determined that he was fit enough to fly home and continue his rehabilitation in the UK. The job was specifically given to me as I had paediatric experience and Alex was, technically, classed as paediatric because he was under eighteen years of age. In reality he was six feet tall and a very sensible young man.

Several delays marred my journey out to Greece to collect Alex. My flight from Manchester was delayed by four hours due to engineering issues which then meant I missed my ferry connection over to the island Alex was on. After a lot of waiting around in the dark I eventually made it to my hotel at four in the morning. I was due to pick Alex up at eight. This wasn't good news for me. I had spent the whole day travelling and could now only catch a couple of hours sleep and a quick shower before heading out again. I also had no time to get a proper meal. But it was what it was so at 7am I was in a taxi on my way to the hospital eating a breakfast of biscuits and a bottle of water – the only fare available from the hotel vending machine.

Sarah and Don had flown on ahead so I was bringing Alex back on my own. We were using the vacuum mattress that mountain rescue teams often use. This is a bright orange mattress that you shape around the patient then attach a pump which removes all the air from it to create a vacuum. When the air is removed the mattress becomes rigid and thus cocoons and protects the patient when they have multiple injuries. The main problem I could foresee was that Alex might get very hot wrapped in this mattress as it was still scorching hot outside and we were heading out into the hottest part of the day.

Alex was predictably pleased to see me but I felt so sorry for him. A big strapping lad with cropped blonde hair, he was virtually helpless with both his arms still in plaster casts and his legs immobilised. He was polite but shy, as are a lot of teenage boys, so as usual I chatted away to him to put him at ease but I did dial it back a little so as not to overwhelm him.

Mindful of the heat and potential mattress issue, I helped change him into cotton shorts and t-shirt and then lined the vacu mattress with a cotton sheet before getting him into it. The nurses kindly provided us with several bottles of water to take with us and I carried out all the pre departure checks: vital signs stable and good; paperwork in order; pain killers given; Alex's possessions packed and ready. Then I sat down with Alex to wait for our ambulance that would transfer us to the airport. 10am arrived and no sign of our vehicle. 10.30am, 11am – still no sign. I asked at the ward reception desk and was told, "It's on its way." But still we waited.

Eventually at 11.30am two burly ambulance men in creased beige uniforms came barging into Alex's room with a stretcher. They ignored us both completely, grabbed the vacu mattress and swung it across roughly onto their stretcher. It was a sign of worse things to come.

Getting Alex into the ambulance, something that should be simple and straight forward, turned into a near disaster. There was no hydraulic platform on the vehicle so the two men just picked up the stretcher and carried it. But the straps they had used to secure the vacu mattress to the stretcher weren't properly fastened. When they tipped the stretcher to enter the vehicle Alex started sliding backwards. Headfirst towards the floor. I grabbed for one of the handles on the vacu mattress and held on for dear life. Luckily, the guy at the back of the stretcher blocked the rest of its fall with his body and between us we managed to hang onto Alex whilst he was loaded the rest of the way into the ambulance. What a pair of cowboys, I thought, hastily checking that Alex was ok. He was, but it was only sheer luck he hadn't hit the floor. I refastened the straps myself once we were safely inside but they were old and frayed: I hoped they would do the job.

"Guess it's going to be an adventure," said Alex giving me a shy grin, his face flushed red and sweat already beading on his forehead.

"Don't worry, it'll all be fine," I replied, returning his grin with a megawatt smile of my own that displayed way more confidence than I actually felt. "We'll have you home before you know it."

The heat quickly assaulted us as the ambulance doors were closed as we were effectively in a tin box in thirty degree sunshine. The two crew, completely unfazed by what had happened, just sat up front chatting between themselves and continuing to completely ignore us. There was a side window; I tried to open it but it was fastened tight. Alex and I shared a look and resigned ourselves to a hot and sticky journey.

"An 'adventure?'" I said. "I think you could be right!"

The drive to the airport turned out to be fast, hair raising and uncomfortable in every way. I was thrown around from side to side as the driver careened around bends at seventy miles an hour necessitating me to hang on for dear life. My seat, of course, didn't have a seat belt so I really hoped that we didn't have to stop in a hurry or I would be in serious trouble. Thankfully the straps on the stretcher held Alex, and the anchor points on the vehicle kept the stretcher in place, but it must have been so uncomfortable for him. His injuries were far from healed and the bone-shaking ride would certainly have been causing him pain. To his credit he didn't complain, just smiled bravely and gritted his teeth. The pain killers I had given him at the hospital were strong ones but in the face of such a white-knuckle ride they were probably having little effect. Several times I leaned forward and asked them to slow down but as we were now running very late they took no notice.

Thirty minutes later we reached the airport and lurched to a halt at the gate that allowed access to the airfield. We waited. And waited. It got hotter and hotter inside our metal box. I gave Alex some water and reassured him that the worst of it was over now. Once on the plane, it would be cooler and more comfortable.

But still we waited.

Then the red tape fun and games began. An airport official threw open the ambulance door and brusquely demanded to see our paperwork. Firstly, he declared our 'Fit to Fly' certificate wasn't completed correctly; then he said our tickets weren't right; then he wanted our passports. It got ridiculous and although I am normally a very patient traveller and am used to hold ups, I found myself getting more and more annoyed. I knew all our paperwork was fine. And I also could tell that although Alex was being very brave, the heat and pain were wearing him down. I tried numerous times to explain that he needed to get out of the heat but my words fell on deaf ears.

We were made to wait again in the ambulance with the doors shut whilst the official took our paperwork to, 'Get it verified'. Many hot minutes crawled by before the door was opened again, this time by two security officers. They said Alex was now to be taken onto the airfield and loaded onto the plane but I couldn't go with him as I would normally do. I had to go through the terminal like a normal passenger. We were to meet up again on the plane.

I was extremely unhappy about this. The idea of leaving Alex alone with these men did not sit well with me apart from the fact that legally, when escorting a patient, I was completely responsible for them at all times. More so with Alex being classed as paediatric. I tried to reason with them explaining that Alex was badly injured and needed me to stay with him and care for him. It was to no avail and eventually I had to admit defeat or we would miss our flight.

Alex had gone pale and an air of panic at being left on his own was swirling around him. I plastered a smile on my face, even though I felt anything but happy at that point, and reassured him again that everything would be okay and we would soon be on the plane and on our way home. It was just the way they did things in this part of the world. I gave him more water and pain killers and made him promise that he would ask for water at regular intervals. We had a bottle left from the hospital so I pushed it down by his side on the stretcher. I waved and smiled at him as I climbed down from the ambulance. Inside, however, I was furious with the security staff and it was taking all my efforts not to have a real go at them. I had learned over the years that doing this is never productive, but gosh, it was hard to bite my tongue that day.

And so it was that I was now sat at the departure gate watching that damn clock, and it was three hours, fifty four minutes and thirty seconds since I had last seen Alex. What on earth was taking so long? The flight was severely delayed now but there had been no explanations given. Several attempts to find out what was going on had been met with the same answer: "As soon as we have any information we will make an announcement."

"But what about my patient? Do you know where he is? What's happening with him?"

"As soon as we have any information we will make an announcement."

I shook my head in frustration.

Six agonising minutes later, thankfully, they started boarding us. I shot to the front of the queue desperate to get to Alex and make sure he was okay. I saw him immediately as I entered the cabin. His stretcher was bolted in place at the back of the plane on the right hand side. I couldn't see his face as he was facing away from me but I breathed a sigh of relief that they had at least loaded him onto the right plane. At that point, I honestly wouldn't have been surprised if he hadn't been there, but on another flight headed who knows where. The airport staff had done nothing to convince me that they knew what they were doing.

I bee-lined straight down to Alex's side. His face was the grey of dirty lace and his eyes were brimming with tears as he struggled not to cry. Sweat coated his forehead and his t-shirt clung to him as if he'd just climbed out of a swimming pool.

"How are you doing, luv?" I asked, dumping my bag on the seat.

As soon as he saw me, his face crumpled and he lost his battle with the tears.

"They just left me," he said. "I didn't know what to do. I was so hot and I couldn't move and my legs were hurting. It was horrible."

It turned out that after I'd left Alex, they had driven the ambulance on to the apron and parked up. A malfunctioning hydraulic lift had meant they couldn't load the stretcher onto the plane until a replacement was found so they had just left him. On his own. In the back of the ambulance. In thirty degree heat. He'd tried to open the bottle of water I'd left with him but his two broken arms had made that an impossible task. When the drivers eventually returned, Alex had asked for water as I'd told him to – they gave him one paper cup full. The bottle I'd left with him was still by his side – unopened. They had barely spoken to him, never once asking him if he was alright or if he needed anything. After almost three hours sitting on the tarmac, the replacement hydraulic lift finally arrived and loaded Alex into the aircraft along with the dinner trolleys and ice cream cart.

Every fibre in my body bristled with anger. The lack of care and compassion was staggering. How dare they treat this boy like that. One thing was absolutely certain: as soon as we were back in the UK I would be putting in a formal complaint.

I immediately set to sponging his sweaty face and giving him a long drink, then rearranged his pillows and adjusted his arms into a more comfortable position. The circulation to his fingers and toes was good and his vital signs were stable – a miracle considering what he'd had to endure. Lastly, I helped him eat some sandwiches I'd picked up in the terminal for him and gave him some more pain relief, all the time chatting away about something and nothing to help sooth his frazzled nerves.

I started to relax a little too: we were back together and Alex was ok. That was the most important thing. But I can't deny that the urge to punch somebody had been very real when I heard about the way he had been treated. Disgusting.

By the time we were ready for take-off, the colour had returned to Alex's face and he looked much more settled. As we levelled off at 35000 feet and the seatbelt sign went off, I glanced over at him and he had fallen into an exhausted sleep. He looked so vulnerable and helpless. Such a young age to go through so much but what a brave young man he was to keep it all together so well.

He slept solidly for an hour. When he woke up he was much brighter and over the next couple of hours I learned a lot about rugby. Alex was hoping to become a professional player and had already been scouted for an under eighteen's team. It was obviously his passion as his eyes lit up when he started talking about previous successes he had had whilst playing for his school team. Several times he had earned the title of 'Man of the Match'. He was also hoping to get a sport's scholarship for university.

But then he suddenly stopped talking and looked away.

"You ok?" I asked.

"I was just wondering if I've messed it all up."

"What do you mean?"

"With all this," he said, nodding sadly at his arms and legs. "I don't know if I'll ever be able to play again."

"What did the doctors say?" I asked gently.

"They said it was doubtful."

"But not impossible?"

"No, not impossible."

"Then you have to hold onto that, Alex," I said. "There's still a chance and you have to try."

He nodded. "That's what my Dad said."

"And he's right, Alex. You've got to go for it."

"Do you really think I can do it after all these injuries?"

"Honestly? I don't know, Alex. But what I do know is you will regret it if you don't try. Just give it your best shot and see what happens."

He nodded again. "Thank you for helping me and for listening."

"It's my pleasure."

Sarah and Don were waiting for us at Heathrow. We were soon loaded into the ambulance – by a very professional and pleasant paramedic crew who were the exact opposite of their Greek counterparts - for the short journey to the hospital that Alex was being admitted to.

After we had been booked in through A&E, I gathered my things ready to leave them. Both Sarah and Don hugged me and thanked me profusely. It was obvious a load had been lifted off their shoulders now that Alex was safely home again.

"He's a good lad, you should be very proud of him," I said.

They both nodded and smiled. "Yes, he is. Thank you so much."

I went back into the cubicle to say goodbye to Alex. Reaching over, I gently squeezed his hand. "Remember," I said, "give it your best shot. With determination like yours, you'll get there. Don't ever give up."

It always surprised me when I was doing these repatriations what a close bond I was often able to form with the patients. Considering we were together for such a short period of time I always felt as if I'd got to know them quite well. And I always cared about what happened to them. Maybe it was because they were so relieved to be going home that they connected more deeply with me as the person who was making that possible; I was keeping them safe when they felt at their most vulnerable. Or perhaps it was because the journey was oftentimes quite intense so we experienced the ups and downs together. And, of course, there was the fact that we had time to talk on a long flight, one of the benefits of working one to one with a patient in this scenario that you don't often get in a hospital setting. It was probably a combination of all these factors but getting to know the patients so well was definitely one of the high points of the job. It was immensely satisfying to know I'd helped them and their families when they most needed it. And I was rewarded many times with cards and updates that made my day when I received them.

Several months later, one such update arrived from Sarah and Don. When I opened the envelope it contained a thank you card and a photograph. A happy Alex grinned at me in full rugby kit. On the back of the photo he had written, 'I didn't give up!'

CHAPTER 15

Red Tape

Most people who travel will have experienced the proverbial 'red tape' at airports. Like with Alex in Greece, it usually means inconvenience and delays but rarely causes any major problems. Occasionally however, it can cause issues that are quite serious. And of course, the more you travel, the higher the probability that a serious red tape problem will get you. I was traveling a lot so it was only a matter of time, and just like buses, two incidents came along virtually back to back. In one, I was nearly arrested as a potential terrorist, and in the other I was refused entry and deported out of the country on the same plane I'd come in on.

No matter how careful you are with paperwork – tickets, visas, Fit-to-Fly certificates etc. (and I quickly learned to be very careful and triple check everything!) – sometimes the problem comes from left field and is totally out of your control.

The first incident happened after I had just landed in Vancouver on the West Coast of Canada. Travelling on my British passport, Canada was a place I had visited several times with no problems. Twenty four hours of exploring stretched ahead of me before I collected my patient so I was in good spirits as I made my way towards passport control. For once the queue wasn't too big so I expected to be through quite quickly.

"How long are you planning to stay?" asked the Border Control agent as he scanned my passport. He looked very young with skin so smooth it suggested he didn't need to worry about shaving yet.

"Until the day after tomorrow," I replied.

"Why are you only staying for 36 hours? What's the purpose of your trip?"

"I'm picking up a patient to escort them home. I'm a nurse."

I wasn't worried. Just routine questions, I thought. As I've already said, I always made a point of being polite and patient when encountering any hold ups. These people were just doing their job; it was nothing personal. And, of course, being bad tempered and inpatient can often have the opposite effect than desired, making things go even slower.

"Can you tell me why you were in Egypt for less than 24 hours?"

"The same reason I am here today. I was collecting a patient."

"And were you collecting a patient the week before when you were in Saudi Arabia for only thirty six hours?"

"Yes, I was, it's my job."

He studied my passport some more, flicking the pages over one by one, examining every detail. I waited patiently. The queue was building up behind me.

After another couple of minutes, he looked up and gestured to an older man in the same Border Force uniform. Obviously his supervisor, this man carried with him an air of authority and confidence. He scrutinized the pages of my passport too and they conferred quietly together for a few seconds. I strained to try and catch what they were saying but I couldn't. Glancing over my shoulder, the queue now wound its way all the way back towards the doors with people shuffling from foot to foot with impatience. A woman with a pram behind me caught my eye and tutted.

The young officer was now clicking away at his computer with the older man looking over his shoulder.

"Is there a problem?" I asked, and then instantly felt stupid. Of course there must be a problem or they wouldn't be holding everything up like this. But I had no idea what that problem could be. Then the older man said, "Can you step to one side, please, Ma'am? We're going to need to do some more checks."

"Yes, of course," I replied, giving him my best 'I am relaxed and not worried' smile. It wasn't returned. Uneasiness started to wriggle around in my stomach. I am one of those people who has never ever been in trouble with 'the law' of any kind – a proper little goodie two shoes – so although logic told me that everything was above board and as it should be, I couldn't help the tingle of anxiety that was creeping over me. Had I inadvertently done something that was going to get me into trouble? I shoved the thought away. It's just routine, don't be so dramatic.

The older officer led me to a room off to the side and I could feel everyone in the queue watching me. It'll be something and nothing, I reassured myself, as I followed him into a windowless room with white painted walls, a metal desk and two chairs facing each other.

The problem turned out to be that I had done several short trips to Middle Eastern countries within the last three weeks. The longest one was forty eight hours – most were quick turnaround jobs of twenty four hours or less. At this time – 2002 – 911 had not long since happened and authorities were understandably being super cautious. They thought it highly suspicious that I was flitting in and out of countries, especially Middle Eastern countries, and literally only staying a few hours. The fact I was travelling with just a carry-on bag and no checked baggage was also raising a red flag. To do such a long journey with just a ruck sack was considered odd.

Sitting opposite the older man across the desk – his name tag identified him as R. Jenkins - I explained again that I was an In-Flight Nurse and what my job entailed. He had never heard of such a job.

"Do you have any I.D. that confirms what you do?"

I showed him my badge.

"You could have made that at your kitchen table," he said flatly.

It was a valid point. The badge I carried was a simple piece of white card with my photo, name and the words 'In-Flight Nurse' printed on it then laminated.

"Yes, I could, I agreed, but I didn't."

He scribbled something on a form he had in front of him on the desk. I waited, noticing for the first time his thick-set arms and the way his shirt strained against his broad shoulders. He wasn't tall – maybe five eight – and looked to be perhaps in his early fifties, but he had an aura about him that suggested it would be unwise to mess with him. I guessed he could be ex-military.

"Do you have a contact number for your company in the UK so that we can check your story?" he said, looking up and holding my gaze with steel grey eyes that weren't unkind but did have an intensity about them that made you want to look away.

'Your story' – gosh, I really was beginning to feel like a suspect in one of my Dad's old Bruce Willis films. But I did, of course, have a number for the office so wrote it down for him.

"Wait here," he said. "I won't be long."

I heard the door lock click as he exited. The tingle of anxiety in my stomach was gathering pace now and making its way up into my head. A banging headache would soon add to my woes. And I was very thirsty – another facet of the anxiety I was feeling – which would no doubt make my headache worse. But I'll be on my way soon, I reasoned. Julie or Tom at the office will vouch for me and it'll all be sorted as quickly as it started.

Unfortunately though, it wasn't.

"There's no answer," R. Jenkins said, when he clicked his way back into the interview room. I sighed with frustration. With the time difference it was the middle of the night in the UK but there was always someone on call for emergencies so they should have answered.

"What about the hospital?" I asked, as he once again sat writing on the forms in front of him. We were facing each other across the grey metal desk, not more than three feet apart. I could smell his musky aftershave and see that the watch he was wearing was a Casio. "I have the number and they will verify that I'm here to pick up one of their patients." He nodded so I scribbled that number down and handed it to him.

Again, he left the room. It really was quite intimidating sitting there in a white room containing just a metal desk and knowing you were locked in. After watching lots of crime dramas on television, I also wondered if someone was watching me although there didn't appear to be any cameras anywhere. There were certainly no mirrors, two way or otherwise. I crossed my fingers and hoped this call would be successful. As is often the case, though, when things go wrong, one thing after another goes wrong. It becomes like a game of dominoes and the whole thing falls down.

That number was unobtainable.

To be fair, he had tried as he had looked up the name of the hospital I had given him and found another number. Unfortunately the person who answered knew nothing about a repatriation scheduled for the day after.

And this time when he came back into the room he had a blonde female officer with him. Polite, business like, but, just like R. Jenkins, not to be argued with. My heart rate raced upwards, thudding in my ears and flushing my face with embarrassment. This could only mean one thing. Thankfully I was spared the 'strip search' nightmare but had to stand with my arms out whilst the female officer patted me down. She then asked for my ruck sack. Its contents were taken out, item by item, laid out on the table and examined. Maybe my stethoscope and other equipment would convince them I was genuine. But they didn't take any notice of it. I suppose if I was 'up to no good' then I could easily have put those items in my bag as cover in the same way as I could have just made my own I.D. badge. It is an odd feeling to watch someone going through all your things. Intensely personal, quite unpleasant; not something I want to repeat too often if ever again.

Four hours had now passed. My headache was banging away like an award-winning rapper and my mouth was sand paper. I asked for a drink and the female officer brought me a paper cup full of tepid water. Then she left. Once again, it was just R. Jenkins and me. We were getting nowhere and I was getting weary.

"What happens now?" I asked, when yet another attempt to

reach the office in the UK had failed.

"Well," he said, leaning back in his chair and holding my gaze again, "we are very concerned about all the trips you have been making to Middle Eastern countries. Unfortunately, until we can verify your I.D. and why you are here we are unable to allow you entry into Canada."

"What does that mean? Am I going to have to sit here all night?"

"No, we will take you to the detention centre and then try again in the morning."

I was mortified. Frustration and tiredness threatened to bring tears.

"Look," I tried again. "I am a nurse, here to collect a patient. I have our return air tickets. Please could you try the hospital one more time? Someone there must know about it and be able to vouch for me."

He sat forward in his chair, resting his arms on the table and folding his hands together. His eyes locked on mine. For a few seconds they bored into to me and then his expression softened and his voice lost its granite edge. "I do believe you," he said. "But I just can't authorise your entry until I have verification."

"Please," I said, "will you try just once more?"

He seemed to be mulling over what to do. Should he try again? Or was he just wasting his time? Then he gave a decisive nod. "Okay. Give me everything you have – Dr's names, ward details – anything."

Twenty minutes crawled by. Then thirty. This was taking too long – it couldn't be good. I resigned myself to a night in a cell, trying to make myself feel better by thinking how much Dad would laugh when I told him. I would be the butt of many a family joke after this and could hear my new nick name 'Wendy, the jail bird' ringing in my ears. But I had done nothing wrong; I was just doing my job. It seemed so unfair. I did have to concede that maybe it looked a bit suspicious but it had just been one of those things that one job after another had come up in the Middle East. It had never occurred to me that it could be a problem further down the line. That maybe someone would think I was involved in terrorist activities, relaying information or acting as a go-between.

Another ten minutes went by. Then another. At long last the door opened and he was back. And for the first time that day he was smiling. Patiently sitting on the phone whilst he was passed from one hospital department to another, his persistence had paid off. Eventually he hit the mark when he was put through to someone who knew about the repatriation. They had confirmed my 'story' and I was free to go.

I was so grateful to him for going the extra mile to resolve the issue there and then. Yes, he had been rather intimidating initially but it was his job to root out potential threats and to keep everyone safe. It was nothing personal. And in fact as soon as he knew I was who I said I was his whole demeanour changed. His brusque tone of voice disappeared and those razor sharp grey eyes even had a hint of humour in them when he said he could still offer me a room for the night if I needed somewhere to stay!

To say I was relieved was an understatement. My passport was stamped and then I 'got the hell out of dodge' as quick as I could. I needed fresh air and I needed coffee. And the toilet! Happily, my 'goodie two shoes' image was still intact but I did feel stupid for getting upset. You need to toughen up, I told myself. You could have had to spend a night in a cell – so what. There are much worse things than that so in the grand scheme of things it was a minor hiccup.

The little bit of free time I'd had had been consumed by this escapade but I made it to my hotel in time to get an evening meal and then some rest before heading to the hospital in the morning. This was the one and only time I had more than just a basic meal on my expense account. I was so relieved to not be sitting in a detention centre that a treat seemed in order; a treat of more than just a sandwich and a can of pop. So I splashed out and had a delicious pasta dish accompanied by a glass of red wine – not exactly fit for a Royal but very enjoyable. Oh, and there may have been a cheeky little piece of Tiramisu as well!

The second incident happened just two weeks later and was altogether scarier and more unpleasant. It also didn't end as well – for me or the patient.

The job, ironically, was to go to yet another Middle Eastern country; this time to pick up a business man who had been in a road traffic accident. A collision with a lorry had written his car off and given him fractures to both legs along with a neck injury – not life threatening but certainly traumatic for him. Normally based overseas, his company had agreed to bring him home to the UK whilst he recovered.

Julie at the office was unable to get me a visa to enter the country: they would issue me with one but there would be a wait of several weeks. Alan, the patient, understandably wanted to come home as soon as possible; he had already been certified by his doctor as fit to fly. After much to-ing and fro-ing with their embassy in London, it was agreed that I could meet and collect Alan in the departure lounge at the airport. I wouldn't officially enter the country so didn't need a visa. The embassy provided a letter stating that I was allowed to go through to the departure lounge to meet up with Alan and then we would leave together. It would be a long day with lots of flying time but I was happy to do it if it meant getting Alan home sooner rather than later.

No one, however, had told any of the officials at the airport about these arrangements. On presenting the letter from the embassy at passport control I knew instantly there would be a problem. A surly middle-aged man with greasy black hair and a moustache was manning the passport desk. He barely glanced at the letter then starting paging rapidly through my passport.

"No visa," he said curtly without even looking at me.

"I was told I didn't need one," I replied. "Your embassy in London gave me that letter – I am only collecting a patient from departures and then leaving again."

His eyes slowly lifted from my passport and his stare sent chills skittering down my spine.

"No visa, no entry."

I explained again what I was doing and about the letter. He

either wasn't listening or didn't understand what I was saying due to a language barrier.

"Could you ring the embassy to clarify?" I asked.

"No visa, no entry," he repeated in a thick, heavily accented monotone that seemed as oily as his hair.

Two more minutes passed as he yet again went through the pages of my passport. I wasn't sure what else to do so I just waited patiently, taking a few deep breaths to ease my creeping anxiety levels. Practically speaking I realised there was little else I could do. I didn't have a visa. They would either accept the letter or they wouldn't.

He looked up and stared at me again. But this time his eyes slid slowly down my body and back up again, lingering pointedly on my chest. His eyes were like knives cutting through me and it was all I could do not to look away. I had heard the expression 'undressing you with his eyes' many times but never before actually experienced it. It was deeply unpleasant. He had such a threatening aura about him. I was glad that we were in a busy airport and not in an isolated room somewhere. I decided to give him a cartoon name to lighten the mood – he would now be Mr Moustache. That is such an original name, I thought, smiling to myself – not!

"Stay there," he barked.

I watched him strut over to the next desk and start conferring with another man. Snatches of Arabic drifted over to me but as I don't speak the language I had no idea what they were saying. Police officers in beige uniforms ringed the arrivals hall – every one of them with a gun on their belt, some also with machine guns slung over their shoulders. A fug of intense heat seemed to hang over me as I stood waiting.

Then my heart fell with a thud as Mr Moustache came back towards me, waving over two of the armed police officers as he did so.

"No visa, no entry," he sneered. "You will come with us." Abruptly, he turned on his heel and walked away. The two police officers, big men who both looked like clones of Mr Moustache with black hair and the same bushy facial hair, moved in behind me and grabbed hold of my arms. With one at each side I was propelled forcefully along behind him. Was this really happening? Surely, things like this didn't really happen. I had given him a jokey name but this was far from funny. I was a long way from home, on my own, and I felt very vulnerable.

I tried really hard to breathe slowly and keep calm. One, two, three I counted. Keep smiling. One, two, three. I was obviously not going to be allowed to collect Alan. The question was what would happen now? Hopefully, I would just be put on the next flight out. I had done nothing wrong, it was purely the fact I didn't have a visa. Surely that wouldn't warrant anything more drastic. But I was thoroughly intimidated with fear gripping me almost as tightly as the two man mountains that had hold of my arms. Their grip would almost certainly leave bruises.

They steered me down a long corridor towards what I hoped was the departure gate for the next flight back to London. But then about half way down they stopped outside one of the doors lining the corridor and I was ushered into yet another bare room containing just a metal desk and chairs. It seemed as if this was standard layout for airport interview rooms. But why did they want to ask me anything? It was a clear cut case of I just didn't have a visa. Mr Moustache had gone in first but the two police officers didn't follow me in. The door lock clicked shut behind me.

To my horror I realised I *was* now alone in an isolated room with this man who radiated an air of menace. It was almost as if the room was charged with electricity as every hair on the back of my neck prickled to attention. I stayed near the door although I knew the other two heavies would be waiting outside so it would be pointless to try and leave.

Mr Moustache turned slowly but this time his eyes were smiling rather than staring - infinitely more creepy and unsettling. A brief image of R. Jenkins back in Canada flashed into my mind. What I wouldn't give to be back there with him rather than here. I was trying valiantly to breathe slowly and keep calm but my heart was thundering in my ears. This was not good. Mr Moustache wasn't moving, just standing there smiling, his brown eyes once again roaming over my body.

Then he stepped forward, moving towards me, his belly hanging over his trousers, threatening to burst his shirt open. Stopped right in front of me. His breath hit my face in little gusts, reeking of tobacco and garlic. Still he smiled, his eyes staking their intent, their desire spilling over onto his fat cheeks. I stood my ground. Held his gaze. Was acutely aware that we were millimetres apart. Then he was moving again. Walking around me. Sidling up behind me.

And then his hands were on me, snaking around me, grabbing at my breasts and yanking me backwards. I tried to break free but his arms were like a vice around me. My breath whooshed from me. The garlic and sweat smell churned up bile in my throat. His fingers were squeezing, twisting, hurting. I felt his mouth on my neck, burrowing in, kissing and sucking, his erection pushing up behind me. Grinding against me. Thrusting and shoving. Then his hands were under my shirt. With a single yank he had my bra up. Twisting and pummelling my breasts. Hard, callous fingers squeezing my nipples so hard it made me gasp in pain. I threw my head back trying to break free but he was so strong. Again and again I tried but still he held me against him, squeezing me so tightly I could barely breathe. My breasts were on fire. My skin burning.

Then I felt his hand move downwards. In one swift move he ripped open the zip on my jeans. Thrust his hand down. His fingers were hot pokers. Probing. Rubbing. Violating. All the time pulling me back, grinding against me. Whispering in my ear as if he thought I should be enjoying this.

Ever nerve in my body was screaming. This couldn't be happening. Blood thundered in my ears as I tried desperately to pull away. Imagined my gentle Dad back home; his hands only ever used in kindness. And then I was dragged me back into that horrible moment as this monster's fingers found their target. I gasped, unable to stop myself from uttering a cry of anguish. No, no, no. I had to get him off me.

With every ounce of effort I could muster I rammed my elbow back into his gut. Powered by rage and horror, it caught him off guard. Gave me a precious second as his grip loosened. I shoved his hands away and wrenched myself free. Raced away from him. Turned immediately to keep him in my sights. Panting. Watching. Ready to fight if he came at me again. Just try it, you bastard. He seemed to be considering doing just that, his smarmy face sneering at me. I saw his yellow teeth, the sweat on his face, that god-awful moustache. The tobacco smell hanging like a poisonous cloud in the room. I felt like a hare cornered by a raptor. If he came at me with any more determination I didn't know what I would do. Except fight like hell.

Abruptly, he seemed to decide I wasn't worth the effort. Within seconds he had turned and was gone. Panting, my heart beating so fast I thought it would explode out of my chest, fighting back tears. Breathe, Wendy, keep calm. He's gone. You're ok. You did it.

But even as those thoughts were registering, the door was opening again. He was coming back. Was he bringing his buddies in to help him? I would have no chance against three of them. Adrenaline burned through my veins. Fists clenched, I braced myself to start kicking and screaming.

It wasn't him.

One of the two heavies stood in the doorway, but made no move to come in.

"Stay away from me," I ground out through clenched teeth. "Don't even think about coming near me." The bravado was false as I was desperately fighting back tears, but I was determined they would not see me as an easy target.

The side of his mouth lifted in a bored smirk and then he beckoned me into the corridor.

Fear propelled me out of the room like the cornered animal that has just seen a chance of escape. They reached for my arms again but I managed to shrug their hands away and set off up the corridor as fast as I could go, straightening my clothes as I went. Thankfully, they just lumbered after me without further intervention.

The corridor did indeed lead to the departure gate and I was so relieved to see there were a dozen or so other people milling around. They couldn't do anything now, not with so many people about. One of the policemen pointed to a seat and I sat down, still watching their every move. One of them spoke in Arabic to a member of the ground crew at the gate and then they just walked off, the guns on their belts banging against their legs as they moved. Just like that . . . they were gone.

I took a few deep breaths trying to hold back the tears and the shock that was simmering very close to the surface. Logic tried to talk me down: I was safe now; what had just happened was little more than a grope; I would soon be on a plane back to London. But, as it would anyone, it had shaken me to the core. I am fortunate to have only ever known good, kind men. Never before had I seen such malevolence in someone's eyes. Someone who could hurt someone else without giving it a moment's thought. We all know evil exists in the world but we also often think these things happen to other people not us. And they certainly don't happen in a crowded airport, in the middle of the day. It was yet another aspect of the steep learning curve that the In-Flight role had set me off on. I had naively been trotting all over the world on my own without giving it a second thought; always careful and sensible, but oblivious to the danger that could be lurking in the shadows. Until today. Today, I had been hit in the face with it. This episode stripped away a large chunk of that youthful naivety like sandpaper stripping away skin, my idealised view of the world well and truly challenged. It was not something I would forget in a hurry.

After a trip to the bathroom to try and wash off some of Mr Moustache's disgusting stench and make myself feel a bit more presentable, I headed back to the gate to see that the crew were now boarding my flight back to London.

Resting my head back against the seat I took another deep, steadying breath. Then the adrenaline crash abruptly overwhelmed me. Up until then I had been on high alert, in survival mode, ready to fight. Now the adrenaline was gone. Every part of my body felt battered and sore, bruised and violated. Dizziness circled around me with its sidekick nausea. And I couldn't stop shivering. Then the tears came.

But there was also tremendous relief. Not only could the 'incident' in the interview room have been much worse, there was also the fact that my paperwork had not been to their liking so I could have ended up being detained further. Thoughts of dark and dank Middle Eastern prison cells crowded into my mind; I was so grateful all they had done was deport me. I had done nothing wrong but sometimes in some parts of the world that doesn't seem to matter. What a total waste of all that time and money though, I thought. All the effort involved in making those arrangements – all for nothing.

Alan had indeed been waiting for me in the departure lounge but he had not been allowed to board because he didn't have a nurse with him. He had been taken back to the hospital. My heart went out to him as it must have been so disappointing to be so close only to then not make it onto the flight. He had to wait another three weeks whilst a visa was sorted and his repatriation rescheduled. I was on holiday so one of the other nurses went. I have to admit I would very likely have said no had it been offered to me.

It turned out that during the Canada episode, there had been a power cut which had taken out the phone back at the office. It was just unfortunate timing that it happened at the moment R. Jenkins was trying to contact them to verify my I.D. and the purpose of my visit to Vancouver.

With regards to Mr Moustache, I told Tom what had happened. He was enraged that one of his nurses had been subjected to that kind of treatment and offered his full support. However, considering that I didn't even know Mr Moustache's real name, and that it had happened in a country thousands of miles away, I decided not to pursue any further action.

I never told my Dad. It was a burden he didn't need to bear.

CHAPTER 16

Nairobi

Sometimes a job didn't end well for other, much sadder reasons. Occasionally, someone would die on the flight home. Thankfully in my career this only happened once, and ironically it wasn't my actual patient.

Although I didn't travel in uniform, the airline always had it on their manifest that I was a nurse. One day, on my way home from Nairobi in Kenya, a member of the cabin crew came over to me and whispered quietly, "We have a very poorly man in the forward cabin. Would you come and take a look at him?"

"Of course," I replied, unbuckling my seat belt and following her. On this particular leg of the trip I didn't have a patient with me so was free to go and help wherever I could. When I did have a patient I had to be mindful of making sure they were cared for before helping anyone else as they were my primary responsibility.

The man they wanted my help with was Ron, a seventy-four-year-old gentleman who was returning home from a two-week safari in the Great Rift Valley. A wedding anniversary gift to his wife, Elsie, they had been celebrating fifty years together. For the first half of the flight he had been suffering terrible diarrhoea and vomiting. A toilet had been made available for his sole use both to help him and in case he had anything other than food poisoning. The crew had provided plenty of fluids for him to sip and he had eventually stopped vomiting and settled down next to his wife for a sleep. Sat in the window seat he was exhausted and had complained of feeling cold so Elsie wrapped him in blankets and an extra jumper. Relieved when the shivers finally stopped and he dropped off to sleep, she too had then nodded off. The cabin lights had dimmed and a hushed quiet drifted down as everyone slept. Elsie had slipped into a deep, weary sleep. An hour later when she woke up, she was unable to rouse Ron. She quickly alerted the cabin crew who then came to get me.

Very sadly, as soon as I removed the blankets and looked at Ron, I knew that he had passed away. Elsie had thought he was unconscious but he had actually died in his sleep. To be certain I checked for respirations and a heartbeat but his skin was mottled blue and already cooling to the touch so I knew he had probably died soon after settling down to sleep. I pulled the blanket back up around his shoulders and turned to Elsie. She was standing behind me in the aisle while I examined Ron. The colour had drained from her face and her eyes were shocked into saucers. It was obvious she knew something was seriously wrong but I don't think that at that moment she had realised that he had actually died.

Sliding out of the seat, I gently took hold of her hand and led her to the galley were we could have a modicum of privacy. Running over in my mind how I was going to tell her, I turned to face her. But I knew instantly I wouldn't have to. I saw the moment reality punched her and she realised what had happened. Her husband was dead. Tears welled in her eyes and her hand flew to her mouth to catch the sobs. At times like these there are no words to be said that will bring comfort. Instead, I just put my arms around her and held her.

The decision was made that Ron would be left strapped in his seat until we landed. I went back and pulled the blankets further up around him to make it look as if he were still asleep. The intention was to try and maintain his dignity as much as possible and to protect the other passengers from becoming alarmed, but a definite sombre air had enveloped the cabin so I'm sure many of them had realised what had happened.

The Captain came back to see Elsie and offer his condolences. He said a few private words to her and then gave her the choice of staying by Ron's side or going to sit in the first class cabin. She chose to sit by Ron's side.

There is an element of deep sadness to think of anyone having to finish a flight with their dead husband strapped in beside them, but Elsie sat in dignified silence and held his hand the whole way back. I guess maybe it brought her some comfort to have those final hours with him. To know he wasn't left alone. That she was with him to the very end.

The crew moved the closest passengers into other seats and I sat on the other side of Elsie. Every now and then she would reach over and squeeze my hand. We didn't talk much and I didn't do anything else. I just wanted her to know that she wasn't alone.

Although it was heart breaking that Ron had died in this manner, there was another element of comfort there for Elsie: the knowledge that together they had just had the holiday of a life time on safari. Side by side the whole time, they had enjoyed an exciting and wonderful adventure. And they had been able to revel in the true and unconditional love that they had for each other. Ron had been happy. And he had been spared the horrors of a lengthy illness that many people have to suffer. Such a precious thing for Elsie to be able to tuck away in her heart along with all her beautiful memories.

As Ron wasn't my patient, and therefore not my official responsibility, the Captain made all the arrangements. A team came on board at Heathrow and took Ron off the aircraft. Elsie and I followed the stretcher and I stayed by her side until he was safely in the ambulance. After the initial flush of tears she had carried herself with a quiet dignity, remaining calm and composed the whole time. As we parted, she hugged me tightly and said simply, "Thank you".

I headed into the terminal feeling emotionally drained. How I wished I had been able to do something to help Ron. Not being able to save him had left me enveloped in a hollow sadness. It is never easy to accept there is nothing to be done. As nurses we are trained to save life, but a large part of the job is also to facilitate a peaceful and dignified ending when no other options exist. I hoped that my actions had, in a small way, contributed to this. And I had helped Elsie when she most needed someone to be there for her. Facing something like this is horrific enough, but to do it alone is doubly difficult. I never wanted anyone to have to do that on my watch. Somehow though, it just didn't feel enough and my footsteps were heavy that day.

My spirits were lifted a little when a week later a beautiful bouquet of flowers and a bottle of champagne arrived curtesy of the airline. A lovely gesture of thanks that I very much appreciated.

CHAPTER 17

Mum

A wild and windy day shooed me back into the house. Bill, our Border Terrier, and I had been walking off the Christmas excess, enjoying the bracing air and exercise. But after our two hour trek, we were both glad to close the front door on the bitterly cold January day and get out of our wet coats. Despite the awful weather, I was feeling positive and optimistic about the year ahead.

The whole ritual of New Year - the fresh starts, resolutions, ideas for new adventures – always galvanised me into action. Some people find these early weeks of the year an ordeal but the idea of a blank canvas to start afresh always energised me and it has long been a time of year that I enjoy. And the planning is as exciting as the events themselves. Great care is taken in choosing a beautiful new diary that I will enjoy writing in, and the year before I had treated myself to an expensive pen that would last me a lifetime. There is always the ritual of a pot of green tea and time set aside to ponder and dream as I write in my diary for the first time – the first blank page a tangible symbol of hope and new beginnings.

And this year was no different. I was looking forward to more In-Flight nursing trips, and was thinking about starting a Master's Degree. There was also something else percolating away: a very ambitious plan to volunteer at Australia Zoo in Queensland for six weeks. This was something I had been yearning to do for a long time and the thought of actually making it happen gave me goose bumps. One of those adventures that really fires you up and makes you glad to be alive. Could I really do it? Taking six weeks off work; the costs involved; the logistics of organizing it – all serious considerations. But sometimes, as the saying goes, you just have to go for it.

Of course, like lots of other people, my resolutions often fell by the wayside. Real life can get in the way and kick even the best laid plans into mush. And that was about to happen now – in spectacular fashion.

Dad was heading out to do a bit of shopping as I arrived home that day so we passed in the hallway. Mum wasn't in her usual spot on the couch but I didn't give it a second thought; I just presumed she was in the kitchen or bathroom. Some years previously, at the age of fifty-seven, she had had a stroke, but she had recovered well, and although slow, she got about well enough.

Heading into the kitchen to put the kettle on I heard the toilet door open and turned just in time to see her falling sideways towards the fridge. Luckily, it broke her fall giving me time to grab for her before she hit the floor. Mum was a small lady – five feet one and seven stone – so I was shocked at the dead weight that landed in my arms.

"I feel funny," she said, as I struggled to get her into the living room and onto the couch. Unable to help me at all, I only just managed to get her there. She was still talking to me but it was obvious that something was very wrong. I laid her back onto the cushions and grabbed the phone to ring Dad's mobile and tell him to come home. Unfortunately he didn't hear his phone ringing and didn't answer.

Mum started to retch and then vomit. Then she lost consciousness, her skin grey and clammy to the touch, her breathing laboured. I needed to ring an ambulance but I was struggling to get her onto her side and stop her choking. Grabbing towels to put under her head, I was just about able to keep her airway patent. Then I was dialling 999.

My gut feeling was firing stroke alarms at me. Her first one had been a haemorrhagic stroke caused by a burst blood vessel bleeding into the base of her brain. Strokes are commonly caused by blood clots blocking off an artery but sometimes they are due to a bleed. This is the more dangerous type, especially if it happens in the brain stem as this is where the mechanism is that controls breathing and other major bodily functions. We had been told first time round that ninety percent of people who have a bleed like Mum's will die there and then. Of the ten percent that survive initially, most of those will have another bleed and die within six months. She had defied the odds and been incredibly lucky to survive. But it seemed like that luck had just run out.

After what seemed like hours of struggling to keep Mum's airway clear so that she didn't choke, an ambulance arrived. I had also finally been able to get hold of Dad but he had not yet arrived home. The paramedics also suspected another stroke. Blue lights cleared the way through morning traffic to Hope Hospital in Salford. Then we were in resus, a clammer of staff busying around Mum, connecting her to machines and oxygen and fluids.

The relative's room overlooked a car park and contained two chairs and a coffee table. In the middle of the table stood a box of tissues. Eventually, the door opened and I knew as soon as I saw the A&E consultant's face that it was bad news. I had been in this situation many times before but always as the one delivering the news. It was very different to be on the receiving end. Everything receding into nothingness except from his face.

"You need to get your family together," he said kindly. "I don't expect your Mum to make it through the night."

He went on to explain that a CT scan had shown that she had indeed had another haemorrhagic stroke. A big one. And it was in the same place: at the base of her brain, in the brainstem.

I rang my brother, Andrew, who by this time was living in Scotland. He got straight on a train to Manchester. My sister, Caroline, went to pick Dad up.

But by some miracle Mum didn't die that night.

What followed was an epic battle as my five-feet-one-inch, seven-stone mother fought like a lion. Pneumonia and urine infections did their best to take her but still she fought on.

I remember sitting on a blue plastic chair in the corridor, waiting as she was being admitted to the stroke unit that first day. A white plastic carrier bag had been pushed into my hands with her clothes in. Looking inside I saw her trousers and t-shirt screwed up into a ball and shoved into the bag. I confess that in my years as a nurse I have done that too - many times. You are rushing around, crazy busy and you don't even think to fold the patient's clothes up – you just push them into a bag for the relatives to see to. But as I looked at my Mum's things, so carelessly screwed up, I was heartbroken. Heartbroken because her things didn't matter. Heartbroken that I too had done that to other relatives. There was no malice there, no intent to cause distress; it was just something that was done because you were busy. I sat there with tears dripping down my face. I vowed there and then to never ever do that again. Such a small thing, just folding up a person's clothes, but it meant so much. When things are so dire, and people so ill, the only thing you have to cling to are those little things so they become so much more significant.

Another thing I realised that day was how little support there actually was for relatives. Everyone is so focused and so busy – there is no time for anything other than caring for the patients. And obviously they must come first. But as I sat on my own in the corridor that day having been told my Mum was going to die, I was devastated and had never felt so alone. I thought later about how much a kind word or a simple cup of tea would have meant to me. How it would have comforted me to not feel so alone, to feel as if someone cared. As with folding the clothes, I vowed then and there to make sure nobody felt like this when I was on duty. From that day forward I have always made time to find the relatives of my poorly patients; to make sure they know my name and that I am there for them as well as their loved one.

It is true that 'being on the other side' makes you a better nurse. The different perspective opens your eyes to the realities of what it's like when it's you watching a loved one suffer; how devastating it is to be helpless to do anything. As a nurse, you're used to being in control, taking action, making things better; not being able to is incredibly difficult. It certainly makes you empa-thise more with people who are having one of the worst days of their lives. You have been there. You have felt the hollowness, the dread of what's coming next. You are no longer just talking the talk; you have lived it. You have had your heart kicked into pulp and left hanging by a thread.

And I think this is magnified ten-fold when it is happening in a foreign country, far away from home and all that is familiar, so perhaps having this kind of understanding is even more import-ant when working in an In-Flight role.

Mum continued to fight on and not only did she beat the odds again by surviving, but twelve weeks later, she was well enough to be discharged to a nursing home to continue her rehabilita-tion.

All my shiny New-Year plans had been thrown up in the air by this point and lay scattered and forlorn like discarded Christmas wrapping paper. None of them mattered. All I was focused on was being there for Mum and Dad. Dad had always been such a strong and steady presence. He kept us going when Andrea died; he looked after us, told those wonderful stories and made us laugh. But that was with Mum by his side. With Mum now in a nursing home, he was on his own, and without her, he fell apart.

Sadly, although Mum fought valiantly, the second stroke rav-aged her body and left her severely disabled. She never regained her mobility so needed a wheelchair and twenty-four hour care.

This ultimately made it necessary for me to re-evaluate every-thing. To rethink the implications and responsibilities of my In-Flight nursing career. The job was everything I'd dreamed of. I loved it. But the reality was that I was away from home for a lot of the time and the working pattern very irregular. I knew when it came down to it that there was no choice. Mum and Dad needed me and they were more important to me than my job. So I made the decision to give it up.

CHAPTER 18

Florida

Florida was bittersweet. It was the first place I had ever flown to many years previously. I loved the vastness of the place, the happy vibes, and the sheer shininess of the water and the sky. But, having made the decision to leave my In-Flight role, it was to be my last repatriation. Quite fitting, as it brought things full circle and gave me a certain sense of completeness. But there was definitely a tinge of sadness. A small doubt lurking at the back of my mind. Was I doing the right thing? I knew I would never get another opportunity to do this again; it was most certainly a once-in-a-lifetime scenario. But I also knew that Mum and Dad needed me. Carrying on and ignoring that was not something I could do. So, as I packed my equipment in my rucksack for the last time, I put it out of my mind and focussed on the job I had to do.

This trip was going to be a little different. Normally I was bringing British people back home to the UK but this time the task was to take an American lady back home to Florida. I would also usually be on my own with the patient, or have just one other friend or relative with us. This time the whole family group was flying back with us on a chartered holiday flight – all seven of them.

As I set off for London to meet up with Connie and her family, I was feeling more than a little trepidation. A lot of eyes would be watching my every move. I was fully licensed and insured for everything I did in this country and on the flight but Tom had told me not to do anything once we landed, to let the receiving staff take over Connie's care when we were on American soil. The company was taking every precaution against getting sued if anything went wrong. This turned out to be a very wise decision.

Connie was at a hospital in London after fracturing her femur – the thigh bone – whilst on a day out along the Thames. She and her extended family were on a three week holiday when Connie had unfortunately slipped on the wet decking of the boat she was on. She had been in hospital for two days and had been told she would need surgery to pin and plate her leg. This she had refused, saying she would prefer to go home and have the operation done there. The doctors considered this unwise but she had insisted. Reluctantly, the orthopaedic consultant had agreed she could fly home. The plan was to again use the vacuum mattress to cocoon Connie and keep her leg immobile and safe during the flight. But the journey would no doubt be painful as she would have to endure being transferred and moved about whilst still having an unresolved fracture of the largest bone in the body. A bottle of Morphine syrup would be prescribed for us to take with us so that she could have regular, strong pain relief.

Euston Station was its usual chaotic self so after leaving the train I quickly shouldered my rucksack and headed down to the tube to make my way across London to the hospital. A private ambulance had been booked to meet me there with two paramedics who would get us across to the airfield where the chartered flight would depart from.

The tube was predictably busy but there were no hold ups so I made good time. Heading towards the main entrance of the hospital, I caught sight of someone waving at me. Jim, one of the paramedics, had spotted me from where they had been parked up waiting. So far, so good, I thought, relieved that I had found them so easily. Jim and I had done an ambulance road trip together once before when he had met me and my patient at Heathrow and driven us up to Glasgow. With his close-cropped silver hair, smart appearance and six-foot-two frame, he reminded me a lot of my first patient, Frank. Striding towards me, there was an air about him that instilled confidence. It had come as little surprise when I had learned he was a retired police inspector. I was glad to see him, and whilst technically a driver rather than a paramedic, I knew we would be in good hands as he was organised and knowledgeable and an excellent driver.

The scene that awaited us on the ward, however, had a chaotic edge. It was instantly apparent which patient Connie was as all seven members of her family were clustered around her bed as if they were trying to form their own little bubble to keep her separate from everyone else. Each one of them seemed to be fussing around and talking away all at the same time. There was noise, laughter, excitement. At 65, she was a grandmother and wife; the group of seven comprised her husband, son, daughter, their spouses, and her two grandchildren who looked to be about nine or ten years of age.

Jim and his crew mate waited outside in the corridor with the stretcher whilst I headed onto the ward. A Philippine nurse named Nan was looking after Connie. She gave me a handover filling me in on what care Connie had been receiving then led the way to the Treatment Room to sign out the morphine ready for the trip. As a controlled drug, it had to be kept in a locked cupboard within a locked cupboard, and then checked and signed out by two members of staff. Once this was done and I had checked through all the documentation we would need, I made my way over to meet Connie and her family and get her ready to leave. We had plenty time for the journey but I still didn't want to hang around as it was a long drive and there was always the potential for traffic holdups to derail our best-laid plans.

The chatter stopped and they all looked towards me as I approached Connie's bed and introduced myself. She seemed in good spirits as we started chatting but there was the familiar tinge of nervousness around the edges that I often saw. Her holiday had come to an abrupt end and she was about to face what would almost certainly be a long and uncomfortable journey so it was not surprising that apprehension had settled around her shoulders.

Her family started talking amongst themselves as I methodically worked my way through the pre-travel observations, but it soon became apparent that one of her female relatives – her daughter – was busy writing away in a notebook. It transpired that she was documenting everything that was happening – as it happened – along with names, times, locations etc. At the same time, her husband, Connie's son-in-law, was photographing everything with a small digital camera.

I sighed inwardly to myself. I always gave the very best care I could to every patient but I was going to have to be ultra-careful that I covered every base on this trip and make sure every detail was documented in my nursing notes. They were obviously looking for anything that they would be able to sue for and wanted written and photographic evidence to support any claims they made. Of course, I could totally understand them wanting the very best care for their mum, but it sadden me to see them more interested in getting clear pictures of everything than actually making sure she was ok. And I have to be honest and admit it was a little un-nerving to feel that people were watching your every move and waiting to pounce if something wasn't exactly to their liking. The claims culture appears to be becoming much more prevalent everywhere now; rather a sad indictment of modern living.

As I got Connie wrapped in warm clothes ready to leave, I realised that she had a mountain of luggage with her including carrier bags full of gifts and a large handbag. Smiling in a friendly but firm way I made it clear to her family that I was there to care for Connie so they would have to deal with all her suitcases. Normally I was happy to help patients with their baggage but officially it was not my responsibility.

When we were packed and ready, Jim and his crewmate, Phil, came in to get Connie into the vacuum mattress and onto the stretcher. This was to be our first hiccup. She refused point blank to let us use the vacu mattress, wanting instead to go on the standard stretcher mattress. Describing severe claustrophobia, she didn't want to feel restricted or trapped. Despite explaining the benefits of protecting her leg, she was adamant she was not going in it so in the end we had to go without it. This was very unwise. She would be moved around a lot in transit and without the rigid cocoon of the vacuum mattress her fractured femur would be subject to a lot of movement. Bone grating on bone. This potentially would cause her great pain. But the patient's wishes were paramount so we had no choice but to go along with what she wanted. I did however make sure to document in my notes very clearly that she was doing this against my advice.

The family were following us to the airfield in a minibus so it was just Connie and me in the ambulance. On her own, she seemed to collapse in on herself, and although I knew this was going to be a tough trip, I felt sorry for her. She told me that they were only three days into their trip when she had fallen and she felt consumed with guilt that she had ruined everyone's long-anticipated holiday. She had also been putting on a brave face and admitted she was in pain and that she thought she'd maybe made a mistake not having her surgery in the UK. Having had pain relief before leaving the hospital, I couldn't give her any-more at that point so instead concentrated on distracting her with chat. I also asked Jim to take it slow and steady which he did with no problem. In the police he had worked in the traffic division – probably why he had got this job - so his driving skills were of a very high standard.

As we motored towards the airfield, Connie told me all about her grandchildren, Amy and Ben, and about the children's ad-venture camp she went to every summer in New England. She worked there as a volunteer teaching the kids to canoe and paddleboard, and loved nothing more than leading a sing-a-long around the big camp fire that roared away every night. It sounded an ideal way to get out in nature and to keep fit and healthy. At sixty five she was retired now but had been a teacher all her life so keeping the connection going with the groups of children she worked with brought her great pleasure. Reliving her last canoeing adventure, Connie's face became animated and the stress lines on her face melted away to reveal youthful skin and shining eyes. Because she wasn't holding herself as tensely, the pain in her leg eased off to manageable levels and she was no longer letting out little screams every time we went over a bump in the road.

The ground staff at the airfield were expecting us so we were waved through the gates with minimal fuss. Under the wing of our waiting plane stood the hydraulic lift that loads the food trolleys and other supplies on board. Jim and Phil got us out of the ambulance and two ground crew efficiently loaded us onto the platform. Connie held my hand as we rose smoothly into the aircraft. I don't know why but I always found it amusing to get on a plane surrounded by the chicken dinners and the ice cream cart and today was no different. I couldn't resist grinning at Connie as we were flanked on our upward journey by two trolleys full of pop cans and crisps.

But then came hiccup number two. As it was a holiday charter flight, it was a relatively small plane with narrow aisles and a lot of passengers closely packed on board in tight rows. Usually, with a stretcher, we would be pre-boarded, but this time they hadn't done that. Everyone else was seated and waiting for us to get Connie secured so that we could depart. The problem was that the stretcher wouldn't fit down the aisle in-between the seats. This meant that the ground crew had to lift Connie above the heads of the other passengers to get her down the aircraft to the row of flattened seats where her stretcher would be positioned. And Connie wasn't a small lady. After much huffing and puffing they finally managed it but today, health and safety would have vetoed this as it was anything but ideal. How those men didn't hurt themselves I'll never know. And this was all accompanied by the click, click, click of her son-in-law as he took one photo after another. He was also making sure to get a face shot of every member of staff involved. Jim caught my eye on more than one occasion as we both acknowledged what he was doing.

With all the jostling involved man handling the stretcher into place, Connie was by this time screaming in pain and feeling sick. I was forced to delay the flight further whilst I gave her more morphine syrup and anti-sickness medication then adjusted her position to try and make her more comfortable. Ignoring the glares from the other passengers, I worked as quickly as I could. Then the Captain came to see where we were up to. Luckily, he was very understanding and kindly chatted to Connie for a couple of minutes as I packed my things away and got seated. Jim and Phil bade their farewells and the aircraft was secured and readied for take-off. An hour and ten minutes late we finally throttled into the sky.

Then came hiccup number three. It turned out that Connie was travel sick and shortly after we levelled off at 35000 feet she vomited back the medication I had given her, including the morphine pain killer and anti-sickness tablet. Luckily, I had Stemetil, an anti-sickness drug, with me in injection form so, screened off by the small privacy curtain, I gave her a shot of this into her thigh muscle. Hopefully, this would work to settle her nausea and she would then be able to keep the morphine down. It didn't. Sadly, nausea continued to plague Connie and two further doses of morphine were vomited back. I was rather irritated by the fact that we had not been made aware of Connie's travel sickness before we left. If she'd told us, I could have brought the morphine in injection form, but, unaware of the problem, she had been prescribed syrup to avoid her having unnecessary injections. Despite my frustration, I did however continue to feel sorry for her. She was certainly paying the price for her decisions as not only was she in pain, but she also had the indignity of vomiting repeatedly in the middle of a plane load of passengers.

In the end, deep breathing and relaxation techniques quelled the nausea but Connie was still unable to tolerate the analgesia. Her fractured femur was agony. Having a long-standing interest in the use of hypnosis/visualisation techniques to manage pain, I asked her if she would be willing to give it a go. She nodded and, with tears in her eyes, quietly said, "I'll try anything."

I laid my hand gently on top of her fractured leg and started to quietly speak. Using a steady, soft voice I guided her into a state of deep relaxation then described warmth transferring from my hand into her leg and that warmth then radiating through the muscles and soothing the pain. I continued for a few minutes, watching the lines on her face soften once again and her eyes slowly start to close. I felt the tension in her leg lessen and the muscles go loose. After about ten minutes the pain abated sufficiently for Connie to fall asleep. The respite for her was a relief, but also, I have to admit, for me. I was relieved for myself that this had worked as I was running out of options to try and really didn't want to have her in pain for the whole of a long haul flight to Florida. Quietly moving away from her side I sat down in my seat opposite her. Connie breathed deeply and steadily, her eyes still closed. Out of the corner of my eye I caught sight of her son-in-law starting to move towards us as if about to take another photo, but by this point I'd had enough. My thunderous look said exactly what I thought and after a brief moment of hesitation he thankfully abandoned the idea and went to sit down again.

Connie slept on and off, punctuated by episodes of vomiting, but she did get through the flight and eventually we began our decent. I remembered the instructions from the office and once we landed, apart from chatting to Connie, I backed off and undertook no further hands-on care.

Which was just as well.

Two paramedics came to off load us from the plane and as the hydraulic lift lowered us down, it suddenly jammed – two feet from the ground. Hiccup number four. As they attempted to wrestle the stretcher off the lift and down onto the tarmac they got the wheel of the stretcher caught on the lip of the platform. The stretcher tipped and for an agonising moment it looked as if they would drop Connie. She screamed and my heart missed a good few beats. Catastrophe was only just averted as they managed to grab the stretcher in time. The two men didn't seem at all troubled by what had just nearly happened. They brusquely righted the stretcher and set off across the tarmac to the waiting ambulance. Neither of them spoke to Connie or me and they were very rough. I think they must have gone to the same paramedic training facility as the Greek crew who I'd had the misfortune of having to deal with when bringing Alex home. Having been keeping my distance to let them do their thing, the subsequent photos would show that I was in no way responsible for nearly dropping Connie. But gosh, my heart went out to her. Today had been a terrible ordeal for her whilst trying to get home and we weren't there yet. We still had the drive to the hospital to do.

The ambulance shook us mercilessly as we sped along the freeway whilst a nasty draught forced its way around the door and chilled us both through to the bone. Connie was weary; she had well and truly had enough. It was late at night, gone midnight, when we finally lurched to a holt outside the hospital.

Things improved markedly from there as the nursing staff were expecting us and took us straight through to a cubicle. Connie was shivering and wracked with pain. I explained about her nausea and vomiting and the subsequent problem we'd had with her not being able to keep the morphine down. They immediately gave her a pain killing injection and wrapped her up in blankets and a duvet. Her family were following us again in a taxi so I waited with Connie until they arrived so she wouldn't be left alone.

Leaning in to say my goodbyes, she gripped my hand tightly.

"Thank you," she said. "I felt very safe with you."

An older nurse kindly showed me to a small waiting room where I could get a hot drink whilst I waited for them to transfer Connie off our mattress. It would need to be bagged up and taken back with me. This was always the least enjoyable part of the trips for me; I prefer to travel light and hated lugging around equipment and mattresses.

Then came hiccup number five, and it was a belter. The television was on in the waiting area and there in front of me flashed news I did not want to hear. A hurricane was heading straight for us and was expected to hit within the next few hours. My heart beat rattled in my ears. A bloody hurricane! I had had the misfortune to be in Baton Rouge once when a tornado came through. It was one of the most terrifying things I have ever witnessed. The whole night was spent without electricity hunkered down in the bathroom at the centre of the apartment I was staying in – the only room with no glass windows. The tornado smashed around me like an enraged demon and I was seriously frightened. In the morning there were cars flipped onto their roofs and trees uprooted; floodwater everywhere. And now I was in the direct path of a hurricane. Julie had booked me into a hotel so I knew I had to get there as quickly as possible so that I could ride out the storm in the relative safety of the hotel building. I was booked on a flight out the next day but knew that that would now not happen.

Waiting for them to sort Connie out so I could package our mattress up and get moving seemed to go on for ever. I tapped my feet, I did deep breathing exercises, I drank coffee but still my heartbeat thundered in my ears. The tiredness didn't help as it had been a very long day. I really needed to get to the safety of my hotel.

At long last I was in a taxi and on my way. It was 4am when I checked in and then finally fell asleep to thoughts of Dorothy and The Wizard of Oz – it definitely wasn't Kansas but there was a very big storm coming just the same.

Howling winds and torrential rain smashing into the windows woke me the next morning. Thankfully the hurricane had been downgraded to a tropical storm but it was still pretty dramatic and I knew I wouldn't be going anywhere that day. As expected, my flight was cancelled. I managed to call Julie. No problem, she had sorted it and I was rebooked to fly home in three days' time.

The storm meant I couldn't go anywhere or do anything so I headed down to the hotel coffee shop. I always made a point, and still do, of having a book with me when I travel. Frustrating delays then become opportunities to quietly catch up on some reading.

So my trip to Florida turned out to be quite the final farewell. I don't know how many of Connie's son-in-law's photos I appeared in – lots I imagine – but I didn't get sued. In fact, a couple of weeks later Julie forwarded onto me a letter that Connie had sent to thank me. Her fractured femur had been repaired and she was progressing well. When we had been chatting, I'd told her that I loved to read so she had also very thoughtfully included a beautiful bookmark that I still have today.

I found out later that the family had indeed started a law suit against the ambulance crew who had nearly dropped Connie when the hydraulic lift malfunctioned. I suppose it was always going to happen that they would sue someone but thankfully it wasn't me. That wouldn't have been the way I wanted my In-Flight career to end. But to be truthful, I don't really blame them for putting in a complaint. The way Connie was man handled by those two crew members was out of order and very unprofessional. I never found out any further details but I hope they were held accountable for their actions.

CHAPTER 19

Endings

Deciding to give up my In-Flight Nursing career was undoubtedly one of the most difficult things I've ever done. So many superb and unusual experiences had taught me a myriad of things I would never learn in a hospital setting and my nursing knowledge and confidence had grown exponentially. The variety of places I had been sent, and the excitement those trips had generated, ignited a deep sense of passion and I had absolutely thrived in the role.

But more profoundly, I had grown on a personal level. The cloak of youthful naivety had been well and truly cast away in favour of the mature, clear thinking mantle of an adult. Issues that had never been on my radar before were thrust into my line of vision. I had confronted painful feelings, desperate sadness, and the horror of what life could throw at you. Child abuse, poverty, grief had all reared their ugly heads. As in any walk of life you had to find a way of dealing with these horrors without letting them consume you. That is no easy task, no matter how old you are. But I had dug deep into myself. Let these things make me stronger rather than break me. Without a shadow of doubt, most roles within nursing would carry such challenges, but the In-Flight role had pushed me to a deeper and more intense level. Just the fact that I was nearly always dealing with these things on my own, and many miles from home, had made me adept at trusting myself and knowing that whatever was thrown at me I could handle.

But, as already said, behind the scenes the job was very different to the glamourous, shiny image it carried with it. Various friends teased about high-flying romances and the five-star life style; those were harmless and good-natured fun. But others had a more sarcastic edge to their comments borne largely I suspect out of jealousy. Accusations were fired at me ranging from being a 'glorified trolley dolly', to a sexually promiscuous member of the 'Mile High Club'; someone who was 'stealing a living' as it wasn't 'proper work'. Whilst I laughed off most of the jibes some of them did strike deep as it was anything but an easy ride. In fact, it could be seriously hard work and extremely tiring. And it carried with it a massive amount of responsibility. Being solely responsible for a poorly patient 10,000 miles from home in a foreign country could be very daunting and stressful. When things went wrong it was all down to me, and that often felt like a very lonely place to be. The one-to-one nature of the role and getting to know my patients so well also had a down side. Empathy flowed to such a degree that it often felt as if I was absorbing their pain and anxiety so that they didn't have to shoulder so much of it themselves. And it seemed to be cumulative. More and more patients meant absorbing more and more difficult feelings and emotions. Gradually, over time, I found the thrilling edge began to wear off and the excitement no longer sustained me as it had done initially. The constant travelling, the responsibility, the difficult emotions began to slowly wear me down and take their toll on my wellbeing.

The decision to stop was driven by the fact that I wanted to care for my Mum, but it was also the right time to put away my rucksack and stethoscope for my own health. I needed to have some quiet time with a more 'normal' job and a steadier pace. Recognizing when you need to slow down and take a break is, I think, one of the hardest things to do. We are all so accustomed to being busy, busy, busy, and when you have an exciting and covetous job it is easy to just get carried along on the thrill factor and ignore the fact that your health is suffering. I guess that maybe taking the time to slow down and recognize what is truly important is one thing the coronavirus pandemic, that we are all battling with as I write this, may have taught us. It may encourage more people to reassess and re prioritise. I obviously reassessed and reprioritised a long time before Covid 19 came along but maybe others can now benefit from a push in that direction and it will be one of the positives to come out of these difficult times.

It also proved to be the right time to leave for another reason.

A short while after I got back from Florida, Dad started to experience breathing problems when out on a walk. At six-feet-two inches and fit as the proverbial fiddle, he regularly covered six to eight miles a days with our Border terrier, Bill, striding out and loving the fresh air. Always one to be active and busy, I think he particularly enjoyed his walks at this time as it gave him respite from the rigors of caring for Mum. His fitness and 'stiff upper lip' mentality learned in the RAF worked against him though. He carried on, saying nothing about his breathing problems. Upper back pain started to knife into him. Still he carried on and said nothing. Next came a cough. Obviously this was more noticeable and after a couple of weeks listening to him, I insisted that he saw his GP. Of course he played it down, telling her it was just a 'tickle' and never mentioning any of his other symptoms. The GP duly gave him antibiotics thinking it was just a minor infection. By the time I virtually frog marched him back to the doctor and bullied him into telling her the full story, it was already too late.

Test after test followed and each one brought progressively worse news: he had lung cancer and it had already spread to his spleen and adrenal glands. He was Stage 4 and terminal. Chemotherapy was not an option as he was too ill but radiotherapy offered some hope of shrinking the tumour in his lung to improve his breathing and make him more comfortable. Every day for three weeks I drove him to the hospital, taking him to the café for a coffee and a piece of cake beforehand to try and make the experience a bit more bearable. But the treatment was arduous and tiring for him. It helped a little but his steady decline continued.

A few days later, on a Saturday evening, I was sat quietly reading whilst he was having a sleep on the couch. He got up to go to the bathroom and the next thing I heard was an almighty thump as he collapsed on the floor. The toilet door was locked so I had to shoulder it open to get to him. He had missed smacking his head on the sink by a millimetre but confusion had taken over and he was rambling and not making sense. I immediately called 999.

Some hours later following a CT scan of his head we were given the news that the cancer had now spread to his brain. All that could be done was medication to try and keep him comfortable. I got him dressed and took him home.

High dose steroids reduced the swelling in his brain and his confusion abated so we had a couple of weeks of relative peace. Trying to make the most of what time he had left, I took him wherever he wanted to go.

A day out to Doncaster to see the Vulcan aircraft in its hanger will always stay in my memory. When in Germany in the RAF, Dad had worked with these magnificent aircraft and they held a special place in his memory, transporting him back to the happy times that we both cherished. Although no longer in service, there was one hangered at the airport in Doncaster that members of the public could visit. I had booked us tickets on a group tour but after explaining how sick Dad was we were given a private tour where we were allowed to walk under the aircraft and look around it on our own. Dad had lost a lot of weight and grown frail but the pleasure on his face that day was a lovely thing to see. For a couple of hours the cancer was gone and he was a young RAF man again. There were souvenirs and coffee as he chatted to the staff about his time working with the Vulcan; they were so good with him and very kind to us.

As usual Dad kept a brave face on to try and protect Mum and me, but his deterioration accelerated rapidly. His GP arranged for him to go into our local hospice for a few days to try and settle his symptoms down and make him more comfortable. By this time he had a mouth full of ulcers, couldn't eat and swollen legs were making it difficult for him to move around.

One day, as I was pushing him around the hospice garden in a wheelchair, his shoulders started violently shaking. Unsure what was happening, I stopped and moved around to the front of him. He was sobbing uncontrollably. Absolutely breaking his heart. I had only ever seen Dad cry once before – the day Andrea died. I held him for a long time in my arms while he cried. I had never before seen a man who wanted to live as much as he did.

The intention of the hospice stay had been to ease his symptoms and get him home again. He never made it. Seven days later at 6.40am on Sunday morning the call came to say that he had deteriorated even further.

"He may rally round again," the nurse said, "but I don't think he will."

The noisy rattling of his breathing echoed down the corridor. I had heard that sound many times before. I knew before I reached his room that this was it.

Even in such a weakened state he smiled when he saw me and tried to crack a joke. My sister, niece and nephew arrived and we sat holding his hand. An hour later he was gone.

I was cast deeply into grief at his loss, but my over-riding emotion was devastation for my Mum. After all she had been through she now had to go through losing her husband of fifty four years; the strong, loving man who had always looked after her and supported her.

The plan that day had been to go and pick her up from the nursing home and take her to see Dad. Instead, my sister and I had to go and tell her he had died. A lump formed in my throat when I saw she was wearing her purple jumper - Dad's favourite. Completely helpless to do anything else she had asked the staff to dress her in that jumper – a simple gesture that carried with it a life time of love. It was a sad day.

A sense of comfort and peace did ease the grief for me in the days that followed though. I had been able to be there for Dad, to look after him and to make his last weeks as happy as possible. He had always been a strong presence in our lives, a good and kind man who looked after and cared for us all. I felt so fortunate to have had that kind of love helping me navigate through growing up; so fortunate to have had a safe harbour to always return to. And so it meant a great deal to me to be able to look after him when he needed it.

It would be a lie to say I didn't miss my flying adventures - I did - but it had been the right decision at the right time. And now, with Dad gone, Mum needed me more than ever.

We had another two years together, Mum and I.

After losing Dad I thought that she would follow quickly. Disability and ill health had destroyed her body and she was frail and helpless. Factor in the grief of Dad's loss and I thought it would be too much for her to bear. But she still had that heart of a lion and she battled on.

Most days I got her wrapped up warm and comfortable in her wheelchair and pushed her into town. We had our favourite coffee shops for cake and coffee when it was chilly whilst on warmer days picnics would take us to our local park. Even when it rained she liked to go out with a rain cape cocooning her and an umbrella fastened to the corner of the chair to keep her dry. I cherished those times together and I think she was happy.

After a while she became too unwell to go out so I brought treats and made coffee for us in her room. Jelly babies were her favourite; I would break them up for her so that she could eat them without choking. Two or three were enough to make her smile. We roamed the plains of Africa together as I re-read all her Wilbur Smith novels to her. She met him once at a book signing and he was a real favourite. My voice soothed her and she would close her eyes and imagine herself under the hot African sun. I guess it was a way of escaping the confines of her body, her mind able to fly free. It gave me great pleasure to fly with her.

We watched our last sunrise together one morning just before Christmas. By this time a morphine pump was controlling her pain; her breathing shallow and sporadic. We spent a little time in Africa as I read about a herd of elephants gathering at a watering hole in the Masai Mara, then I settled back in my chair and held her hand.

Life after Mum died was a real struggle. It seemed that everything had become about loss. I had lost my Mum, my Dad and my In-Flight career. Giving up my job had meant I could be there for my parents as I wanted to be, and I was so grateful for that, but I did mourn its loss acutely. It had become such a part of who I was. Emptiness soaked into me and weighed me down. Each day became an ordeal, something I had to just get through. There didn't seem to be any bright spots, just the blackness of grief and depression. Everyone else moved on. The world kept turning. But I was stuck. What would I do now?

Grief counselling helped. It took every ounce of my courage to admit that for once it was me that needed the help. I was so used to caring for everyone else and being the person that other people turned to. And it was not only the loss of Mum and Dad that hit me. An accumulation of all the pain and suffering I had absorbed from my patients over the years also conspired to bring me down. Slowly but surely it had stealthily built up around the corners of my psyche. The death of my Mum and Dad was the tipping point, the final straw. There was no more room – I had to let things go and make space for myself. A kind and skilled hospice counsellor helped me to do this. To see that it was time for change. This part of my life had come to a close. I had many precious memories tucked safely away but it was time for a new beginning. A fresh start.

EPILOGUE

The sun is lowering on the horizon and infusing the whole sky with a golden glow that soothes me. The swifts and swallows are back.

I am in the garden amongst my Mum's flowers; they are mine now. A blanket around my shoulders warms me as an evening chill settles. Above my head, the swifts race against the gathering dusk, their wings scything through the air as they twirl and tumble with abandon. Time has moved on but they are a constant, an invisible thread that connects me to all that has gone before. It feels good to sit here whilst my mind wanders around.

I eventually got to Australia Zoo in Queensland. Volunteering there for a few weeks, Kangaroo poo became the focus of my days but I also got to hang out with a koala named Edna, a multitude of wallabies and a litter of five dingo puppies. I also got to witness the wonder that was Steve Irwin, the famed Crocodile Hunter who owned Australia Zoo. His 'rock-star' status was something quite beyond anything I could ever have imagined.

On my first day, an almighty roaring noise erupted behind me and then he shot out of the bushes on a motorbike closely followed by at least a hundred screaming women. As he flew by he shouted, "Strewth, if these Sheila's catch me I'm a goner!" As a volunteer we were often tasked with forming a human security shield around him when he was getting ready to do one of his croc displays. Arm in arm we would create a barrier to keep him from getting mobbed; of course a great advantage to this was that we had a ring side seat to watch him in action which was quite something. Charisma and character oozed from his strapping six-feet-plus frame and he was exactly the same in real life as he was on the television: larger than life, a real giant of a man in every sense. Such a shame that he died the way he did some years later: a freak accident where he was shot through the heart by a stingray barb. I feel incredibly privileged to have met him and been able to see him in action.

Sydney also welcomed me back and I was lucky enough to be able to spend some time there soaking up all the things I had not had chance to do when I was on a job. And it was nice to fly long haul without having to work.

And in case you're wondering, I never did go back to Antigua to marry Uncle Duncan and live with his mum and Elvis the donkey – flattered though I was to have been asked!

Career wise, the winds of change propelled me on. After thirty years of caring for people as a nurse, I hung up my stethoscope for good. It felt strange and surreal as nursing was all I had ever known since starting work; it was who I was. But I am a great believer in taking the leap and seeing what happens. Relishing the adventure and the excitement as I had done all those years ago sat at our kitchen table travelling the world with my Dad and his stories. Courage was one of his lasting gifts. So I swallowed my fears, of which there were a few, and went for it anyway, embracing a new direction and setting up my own business to see where it would take me.

Flying is still a passion and always will be. The moment the wheels of the aircraft leave the runway still gives me a thrilling shiver just as it did when I flew for the first time. Being above the clouds is freedom. Free of the earth, free of boundaries, free to just be. Maybe one day soon I will have a go at getting my pilot's license.

Of course, I still love caring for people. It is in my genes, part of the fabric of my makeup. That will never change. Nursing for thirty years was hard work with many challenges, but it afforded me such wonderful opportunities that I will always be grateful for: meeting a whole cast of fascinating people; travelling the world; adrenaline fuelled adventures. But most importantly it gave me the means to help people when they needed it most; to make a difference, even if only in a small way.

And I will always remember watching Mum stroking Andrea's face and singing to her. Teaching me by example to do little things with great love. That was her lasting gift to me.

So my trusty purple rucksack and stethoscope are still there, hanging safely in my wardrobe. They are a tangible reminder of all the places I've been and the things I've done. Who knows, maybe one day I will use them again.

But for now, I will soar through the sky with the swifts and swallows, dreaming of things to come.

ABOUT THE AUTHOR

Wendy Seddon

Wendy Seddon lives in Leigh, Greater Manchester. After many years spent nursing, she now runs her own business. Her passions are travelling, flying, walking and dogs.

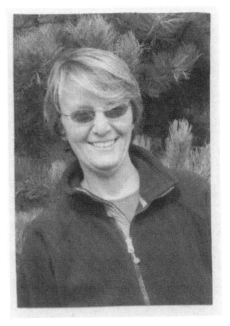

Printed in Great Britain
by Amazon

63724905R00115